AIDS/HIV

ISSN 1532-2718

AIDS/HIV

Brian Hoyle

INFORMATION PLUS® REFERENCE SERIES
Formerly Published by Information Plus, Wylie, Texas

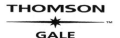

Detroit • New York • San Francisco • San Diego • New Haven, Conn. • Waterville, Maine • London • Munich

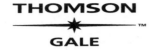

AIDS/HIV
Brian Hoyle
Paula Kepos, Series Editor

Project Editor
John McCoy

Permissions
Margaret Abendroth, Edna Hedblad,
Emma Hull

Composition and Electronic Prepress
Evi Seoud

Manufacturing
Drew Kalasky

ISBN 0-7876-5103-6 (set)
ISBN 1-4144-0404-2
ISSN 1532-2718

This title is also available as an e-book.
ISBN 1-4144-1043-3 (set)
Contact your Thomson Gale sales representative for ordering information.

Printed in the United States of America
10 9 8 7 6 5 4 3 2 1

TABLE OF CONTENTS

AIDS, increased knowledge and tolerance, teen attitudes, and persistence of misinformation about HIV/AIDS. Poll data on the health and well-being of those with HIV/AIDS are also included.

PREFACE

AIDS/HIV is part of the *Information Plus Reference Series*. The purpose of each volume of the series is to present the latest facts on a topic of pressing concern in modern American life. These topics include today's most controversial and most studied social issues: abortion, capital punishment, care for the elderly, crime, the environment, health care, immigration, minorities, national security, social welfare, women, youth, and many more. Although written especially for the high school and undergraduate student, this series is an excellent resource for anyone in need of factual information on current affairs.

By presenting the facts, it is Thomson Gale's intention to provide its readers with everything they need to reach an informed opinion on current issues. To that end, there is a particular emphasis in this series on the presentation of scientific studies, surveys, and statistics. These data are generally presented in the form of tables, charts, and other graphics placed within the text of each book. Every graphic is directly referred to and carefully explained in the text. The source of each graphic is presented within the graphic itself. The data used in these graphics are drawn from the most reputable and reliable sources, in particular from the various branches of the U.S. government and from major independent polling organizations. Every effort has been made to secure the most recent information available. The reader should bear in mind that many major studies take years to conduct, and that additional years often pass before the data from these studies are made available to the public. Therefore, in many cases the most recent information available in 2006 dated from 2003 or 2004. Older statistics are sometimes presented as well if they are of particular interest and no more recent information exists.

Although statistics are a major focus of the *Information Plus Reference Series*, they are by no means its only content. Each book also presents the widely held positions and important ideas that shape how the book's subject is discussed in the United States. These positions are explained in detail and, where possible, in the words of their proponents. Some of the other material to be found in these books includes: historical background; descriptions of major events related to the subject; relevant laws and court cases; and examples of how these issues play out in American life. Some books also feature primary documents or have pro and con debate sections giving the words and opinions of prominent Americans on both sides of a controversial topic. All material is presented in an evenhanded and unbiased manner; the reader will never be encouraged to accept one view of an issue over another.

HOW TO USE THIS BOOK

The spread of AIDS has become a global epidemic. As of 2004 about thirty-nine million people worldwide were living with HIV. Approximately three million people died of AIDS that year. This book provides a snapshot of AIDS/HIV. Included is information on the nature of AIDS/HIV and the AIDS epidemic; symptoms and transmittal; populations at risk; children, adolescents, and AIDS/HIV; AIDS/HIV and the health-care system; cost, treatment, and research; testing, prevention, and education; HIV and AIDS worldwide; and knowledge, behavior, and opinions of those affected by AIDS/HIV.

AIDS/HIV consists of ten chapters and three appendices. Each of the chapters is devoted to a particular aspect of AIDS/HIV. For a summary of the information covered in each chapter, please see the synopses provided in the Table of Contents at the front of the book. Chapters generally begin with an overview of the basic facts and background information on the chapter's topic, then proceed to examine subtopics of particular interest. For example, Chapter Two: Definition, Symptoms, and Transmittal begins with definitions of AIDS and HIV and an explanation of the 1993 classification revision and expanded surveillance case definition. It then goes on to provide information about the diagnosis and symptoms of the disease, its transmission, safety of blood and transplant procedures, and testing for HIV (including diagnostic, urine, and home tests). Readers can find their way through a chapter by looking for the section and subsection headings, which are clearly set off from the text. They can also refer to the book's extensive index if they already know what they are looking for.

Statistical Information

The tables and figures featured throughout *AIDS/HIV* will be of particular use to the reader in learning about this issue. These tables and figures represent an extensive collection of the most recent and important statistics on AIDS/HIV and related issues—for example, graphics in the book cover clinical categories of AIDS infection; adult and adolescent HIV infection and AIDS cases; pediatric AIDS cases; office visits, by diagnostic and screening services ordered or provided; distribution of the number of patients assisted in suicide; syringe exchange statistics; states with confidential HIV reporting; and teens' concerns about becoming infected with HIV/AIDS. Thomson Gale believes that making this information available to the reader is the most important way in which we fulfill the goal of this book: to help readers to understand the issues and controversies surrounding AIDS/HIV in the United States and to reach their own conclusions.

Each table or figure has a unique identifier appearing above it, for ease of identification and reference. Titles for the tables and figures explain their purpose. At the end of each table or figure, the original source of the data is provided.

In order to help readers understand these often complicated statistics, all tables and figures are explained in the text. References in the text direct the reader to the relevant statistics. Furthermore, the contents of all tables and figures are fully indexed. Please see the opening section of the Index at the back of this volume for a description of how to find tables and figures within it.

Appendices

In addition to the main body text and images, *AIDS/HIV* has three appendices. The first is the Important Names and Addresses directory. Here the reader will find contact information for a number of government and private organizations that can provide further information on AIDS/HIV. The second appendix is the Resources section, which can also assist the reader in conducting his or her own research. In this section the author and editors of *AIDS/HIV* describe some of the sources that were most useful during the compilation of this book. The final appendix is the detailed Index, which facilitates reader access to specific topics in this book.

ADVISORY BOARD CONTRIBUTIONS

The staff of Information Plus would like to extend its heartfelt appreciation to the Information Plus Advisory Board. This dedicated group of media professionals provides feedback on the series on an ongoing basis. Their comments allow the editorial staff who work on the project to make the series better and more user-friendly. Our top priority is to produce the highest-quality and most useful books possible, and the Advisory Board's contributions to this process are invaluable.

The members of the Information Plus Advisory Board are:

- Kathleen R. Bonn, Librarian, Newbury Park High School, Newbury Park, California

- Madelyn Garner, Librarian, San Jacinto College— North Campus, Houston, Texas

- Anne Oxenrider, Media Specialist, Dundee High School, Dundee, Michigan

- Charles R. Rodgers, Director of Libraries, Pasco-Hernando Community College, Dade City, Florida

- James N. Zitzelsberger, Library Media Department Chairman, Oshkosh West High School, Oshkosh, Wisconsin

COMMENTS AND SUGGESTIONS

The editors of the *Information Plus Reference Series* welcome your feedback on *AIDS/HIV*. Please direct all correspondence to:

Editors
Information Plus Reference Series
27500 Drake Rd.
Farmington Hills, MI 48331-3535

CHAPTER 1
THE NATURE OF HIV/AIDS

Acquired immune deficiency syndrome (AIDS) is the late stage of an infection that is generally acknowledged to be caused by the human immunodeficiency virus (HIV). HIV is a retrovirus that attacks and destroys certain white blood cells. The targeted destruction weakens the body's immune system and makes the infected person susceptible to infections and diseases that ordinarily would not be life threatening. AIDS is considered a blood-borne, sexually transmitted disease because HIV is spread through contact with blood, semen, or vaginal fluids from an infected person.

Before 1981 AIDS was virtually unknown in the United States. In that year, testing of blood and other samples for HIV began, and reporting of the disease became mandatory. Awareness grew as the annual number of diagnosed cases and deaths steadily increased. By October 1995 the number of U.S. AIDS cases reported since 1981 reached the half-million mark. Indeed, in 1995 HIV infection was the leading cause of death among Americans age twenty-five to forty-four.

By 1998, however, HIV/AIDS deaths among this age group had fallen dramatically, and HIV infection was the fifth most common cause of death among people in the United States between twenty-five and forty-four years old. HIV/AIDS deaths fell to sixth place in the 2001 summary. This rank was maintained in the 2003 summary, with the disease claiming a reported 6,879 lives of the 33,022 total cases of infection. (See Table 1.1.)

On the other hand, HIV as a cause of death increased in those age fifteen to twenty-four between 2000 (178 deaths) and 2001 (227 deaths). But in the 2003 summary the number of deaths in this age group had declined to 171. Reflecting this decline, HIV infection was the seventh most common cause of death in this age group in 2001 and the tenth in 2003. (See Table 1.1.)

Overall, HIV death rates began to decline in 1996, even prior to the widespread use of new and effective drug treatments such as protease inhibitors. In 1997 HIV infection was the fourteenth-leading cause of death overall in the United States. By 1999 HIV infection no longer ranked among the fifteen leading causes of death in the United States. This trend continued in 2000, 2001, and 2003. (See Table 1.2.)

When examined at a general level, the decline in HIV/AIDS deaths between 1995 and 2000 seemed to indicate a positive trend for sufferers of the disease. But the reality was that the actual number of people living with HIV/AIDS increased between 1995 and 2000. In other words, while not as many people were dying of AIDS, more people were living with the disease, due to the success of new therapies. These people will eventually need additional treatment and care.

The observed decline in HIV/AIDS deaths is no reassurance to the estimated forty thousand people who acquire an HIV infection each year in the United States. Furthermore, the Centers for Disease Control and Prevention (CDC), headquartered in Atlanta, Georgia, estimates that one-quarter of the 850,000 to 950,000 people living with HIV in the United States are unaware of their infection.

Despite the overall decline in the death rate, in 1997 HIV remained a leading cause of death for African-Americans age twenty-five to forty-four. By 1999 this death rate was nearly eleven times higher than for white Americans, according to the CDC. African-Americans accounted for 49% of AIDS deaths in 1999 and 51% in 2000, despite representing only 13% of the U.S. population in both years.

The dramatic 42% decline in AIDS deaths between 1996 and 1997 was the result of the introduction and use of effective antiretroviral drugs that slow the progression

TABLE 1.1

Deaths and death rates for the 10 leading causes of death in specified age groups, preliminary 2003

[Data are based on a continuous file of records received from the states. Rates are per 100,000 population in specified group. Figures are based on weighted data rounded to the nearest individual, so categories may not add to totals or subtotals.]

Rank[a]	Cause of death and age	Number	Rate
All ages[b]			
. . .	All causes	2,443,930	840.4
1	Diseases of heart	684,462	235.4
2	Malignant neoplasms	554,643	190.7
3	Cerebrovascular diseases	157,803	54.3
4	Chronic lower respiratory diseases	126,128	43.4
5	Accidents (unintentional injuries)	105,695	36.3
. . .	Motor vehicle accidents	44,059	15.2
. . .	All other accidents	61,636	21.2
6	Diabetes mellitus	73,965	25.4
7	Influenza and pneumonia	64,847	22.3
8	Alzheimer's disease	63,343	21.8
9	Nephritis, nephrotic syndrome and nephrosis	42,536	14.6
10	Septicemia	34,243	11.8
. . .	All other causes	536,265	184.4
1–4 years			
. . .	All causes	4,911	31.1
1	Accidents (unintentional injuries)	1,679	10.6
. . .	Motor vehicle accidents	591	3.7
. . .	All other accidents	1,088	6.9
2	Congenital malformations, deformations and chromosomal abnormalities	514	3.3
3	Malignant neoplasms	383	2.4
4	Assault (homicide)	342	2.2
5	Diseases of heart	186	1.2
6	Influenza and pneumonia	151	1.0
7	Septicemia	82	0.5
8	Certain conditions originating in the perinatal period	76	0.5
9	In situ neoplasms, benign neoplasms and neoplasms of uncertain or unknown behavior	53	0.3
10	Chronic lower respiratory diseases	47	0.3
. . .	All other causes	1,398	8.9
5–14 years			
. . .	All causes	6,930	16.9
1	Accidents (unintentional injuries)	2,561	6.3
. . .	Motor vehicle accidents	1,592	3.9
. . .	All other accidents	970	2.4
2	Malignant neoplasms	1,060	2.6
3	Congenital malformations, deformations and chromosomal abnormalities	370	0.9
4	Assault (homicide)	310	0.8
5	Intentional self-harm (suicide)	255	0.6
6	Diseases of heart	252	0.6
7	Influenza and pneumonia	134	0.3
8	Chronic lower respiratory diseases	107	0.3
9	Septicemia	77	0.2
10	In situ neoplasms, benign neoplasms and neoplasms of uncertain or unknown behavior	76	0.2
. . .	All other causes	1,728	4.2

TABLE 1.1

Deaths and death rates for the 10 leading causes of death in specified age groups, preliminary 2003 [CONTINUED]

[Data are based on a continuous file of records received from the states. Rates are per 100,000 population in specified group. Figures are based on weighted data rounded to the nearest individual, so categories may not add to totals or subtotals.]

Rank[a]	Cause of death and age	Number	Rate
15–24 years			
. . .	All causes	33,022	80.1
1	Accidents (unintentional injuries)	14,966	36.3
. . .	Motor vehicle accidents	10,857	26.3
. . .	All other accidents	4,109	10.0
2	Assault (homicide)	5,148	12.5
3	Intentional self-harm (suicide)	3,921	9.5
4	Malignant neoplasms	1,628	4.0
5	Diseases of heart	1,083	2.6
6	Congenital malformations, deformations and chromosomal abnormalities	425	1.0
7	Influenza and pneumonia	216	0.5
8	Cerebrovascular diseases	204	0.5
9	Chronic lower respiratory diseases	172	0.4
10	Human immunodeficiency virus (HIV) disease	171	0.4
. . .	All other causes	5,088	12.3
25–44 years			
. . .	All causes	128,924	153.0
1	Accidents (unintentional injuries)	27,844	33.1
. . .	Motor vehicle accidents	13,582	16.1
. . .	All other accidents	14,261	16.9
2	Malignant neoplasms	19,041	22.6
3	Diseases of heart	16,283	19.3
4	Intentional self-harm (suicide)	11,251	13.4
5	Assault (homicide)	7,367	8.7
6	Human immunodeficiency virus (HIV) disease	6,879	8.2
7	Chronic liver disease and cirrhosis	3,288	3.9
8	Cerebrovascular diseases	3,004	3.6
9	Diabetes mellitus	2,662	3.2
10	Influenza and pneumonia	1,337	1.6
. . .	All other causes	29,968	35.6
45–64 years			
. . .	All causes	437,058	636.1
1	Malignant neoplasms	144,936	211.0
2	Diseases of heart	101,713	148.0
3	Accidents (unintentional injuries)	23,669	34.5
. . .	Motor vehicle accidents	9,891	14.4
. . .	All other accidents	13,778	20.1
4	Diabetes mellitus	16,326	23.8
5	Cerebrovascular diseases	15,971	23.2
6	Chronic lower respiratory diseases	15,409	22.4
7	Chronic liver disease and cirrhosis	13,649	19.9
8	Intentional self-harm (suicide)	10,057	14.6
9	Human immunodeficiency virus (HIV) disease	5,917	8.6
10	Septicemia	5,827	8.5
. . .	All other causes	83,584	121.7

of HIV infection. This decline continued but slowed to 20% between 1997 and 1998, and only 8% between 1998 and 1999. This may be due to a combination of several factors: resistance to the drug treatments has developed in some patients, the complicated drug treatment regimens can be difficult for patients to maintain, and there can be a lack of access to prompt testing or treatment. According to the CDC, an estimated 929,566 people in the United States had been diagnosed with AIDS up to December 2003. Of these, 524,060 had died ("Basic Statistics," http://www.cdc.gov/hiv/stats.htm).

The AIDS epidemic is by no means strictly a U.S. phenomenon. Researchers for the Joint United Nations Program on HIV/AIDS and the World Health Organization report that AIDS has become a global epidemic that exceeds predictions made in the mid-1990s by 50%.

TABLE 1.1

Deaths and death rates for the 10 leading causes of death in specified age groups, preliminary 2003 [CONTINUED]

[Data are based on a continuous file of records received from the states. Rates are per 100,000 population in specified group. Figures are based on weighted data rounded to the nearest individual, so categories may not add to totals or subtotals.]

Rank[a]	Cause of death and age	Number	Rate
	65 years and over		
. . .	All causes	1,804,131	5,022.8
1	Diseases of heart	564,204	1,570.8
2	Malignant neoplasms	387,475	1,078.7
3	Cerebrovascular diseases	138,397	385.3
4	Chronic lower respiratory diseases	109,199	304.0
5	Alzheimer's disease	62,707	174.6
6	Influenza and pneumonia	57,507	160.1
7	Diabetes mellitus	54,770	152.5
8	Nephritis, nephrotic syndrome and nephrosis	35,392	98.5
9	Accidents (unintentional injuries)	33,976	94.6
. . .	Motor vehicle accidents	7,379	20.5
. . .	All other accidents	26,597	74.0
10	Septicemia	26,609	74.1
. . .	All other causes	333,895	929.6
. . .	Category not applicable.		

[a]Rank based on number of deaths.
[b]Includes deaths under 1 year of age.
Note: Data are subject to sampling or random variation.

SOURCE: Donna L. Hoyert, Hsiang-Ching Kung, and Betty L. Smith, "Table 7. Deaths and Death Rates for the 10 Leading Causes of Death in Specified Age Groups: United States, Preliminary 2003," in "Deaths: Preliminary Data for 2003," *National Vital Statistics Reports*, vol. 53, no. 15, Centers for Disease Control and Prevention, National Center for Health Statistics, February 28, 2005, http://www.cdc.gov/nchs/data/nvsr/nvsr53/nvsr53_15.pdf (accessed July 18, 2005)

According to the December 2004 *AIDS Epidemic Update* (http://www.unaids.org/wad2004/EPIupdate2004_html_en/epi04_00_en.htm), 39.4 million people worldwide were then living with HIV/AIDS. In 2004 alone, an estimated 4.9 million people became infected and 3.1 million people worldwide died of AIDS. The countries of sub-Saharan Africa continued to have the world's highest annual rates of HIV infection and deaths in 2004.

THE HUMAN IMMUNODEFICIENCY VIRUS

A virus is a tiny infectious agent composed of genes surrounded by a protective coating. Until a virus contacts a host cell, it is essentially an inert bag of genetic material. Viruses are parasites. They must invade other cells and commandeer the host cell's replication machinery in order to reproduce. A frequent outcome of viral infection is the destruction of the host cell, as the newly made virus particles burst out of the cell. The host cell destruction can harm the host (in the case of HIV, a human). The common cold, influenza (flu), and some forms of pneumonia are also caused by specific, non-HIV viruses.

HIV belongs to a group of viruses known as retroviruses. The name arises from the presence of a special enzyme—reverse transcriptase—that reverses the usual pattern of translating the genetic message. (See Figure 1.1.) In animals the genetic units of information that are called genes are made up of deoxyribonucleic acid (DNA). DNA is the blueprint from which another type of genetic material called ribonucleic acid (RNA) is made, in a process called transcription. The RNA in turn serves as the blueprint for the various proteins that are the structural building blocks of the virus. In contrast to animals, retroviruses have their genes stored in RNA. After HIV infects a human cell, the viral reverse transcriptase works to transcribe HIV RNA into DNA. The viral DNA then becomes part of the host DNA—a process called integration—and is replicated along with the host DNA to produce new HIV particles.

Prior to 1980 retroviruses had been found in some animals. Indeed, as far back as 1911 Peyton Rous isolated an infectious and debilitating virus from a chicken. The Rous sarcoma virus was later shown to be both an oncogenic (cancer-causing) virus and the first known retrovirus. The first human retroviruses, human T cell leukemia virus (HTLV-I) and the very closely related human T cell lymphotropic virus (HTLV-II), were discovered in 1980 by Robert Gallo and his colleagues at the U.S. National Cancer Institute (NCI). This breakthrough provided the groundwork for the discovery of the virus that would eventually be known as HIV.

Identifying the Virus

In September 1983 Luc Montagnier and researchers at the Pasteur Institute in Paris, France, isolated and identified a retrovirus they named lymphadenopathy-associated virus (LAV). Eight months later Gallo's group at NCI isolated the same virus in AIDS patients, which they called HTLV-III. LAV and HTLV-III were found to be identical and are now referred to as HIV. A conflict arose about which researcher should be credited with the discovery. In 1991, in an intense, politically charged atmosphere, Gallo dropped his claim to the discovery of HIV.

The Origins of the Virus

It has long been speculated that HIV evolved from simian immunodeficiency virus (SIV), a retrovirus that infects monkeys. The theory is that HIV evolved from a human infection with a mutated form of SIV that was infectious to humans. Consistent with this theory is the finding that HIV is a part of the lentivirus family, which includes SIV.

In 1982 Isao Miyoshi of Kochi University in Japan identified an HTLV-related virus in Japanese macaque monkeys. Genetically similar to HTLV, it was designated as the simian T-lymphotropic virus (STLV). Further studies identified STLV in both Asian and

TABLE 1.2

Deaths and death rates and age-adjusted death rates and percent changes for the 15 leading causes of death, final 2002 and preliminary 2003

[Data are based on a continuous file of records received from the states. Rates are per 100,000 population; age-adjusted rates per 100,000 U.S. standard population based on the year 2000 standard. Figures for 2003 are based on weighted data rounded to the nearest individual, so categories may not add to totals.]

| Rank* | Cause of death | Number | Death rate | Age-adjusted death rate | | |
				2003	2002	Percent change
. . .	All causes	2,443,930	840.4	831.2	845.3	−1.7
1	Diseases of heart	684,462	235.4	232.1	240.8	−3.6
2	Malignant neoplasms	554,643	190.7	189.3	193.5	−2.2
3	Cerebrovascular diseases	157,803	54.3	53.6	56.2	−4.6
4	Chronic lower respiratory diseases	126,128	43.4	43.2	43.5	−0.7
5	Accidents (unintentional injuries)	105,695	36.3	36.1	36.9	−2.2
6	Diabetes mellitus	73,965	25.4	25.2	25.4	−0.8
7	Influenza and pneumonia	64,847	22.3	21.9	22.6	−3.1
8	Alzheimer's disease	63,343	21.8	21.4	20.2	5.9
9	Nephritis, nephrotic syndrome and nephrosis	42,536	14.6	14.5	14.2	2.1
10	Septicemia	34,243	11.8	11.7	11.7	—
11	Intentional self-harm (suicide)	30,642	10.5	10.5	10.9	−3.7
12	Chronic liver disease and cirrhosis	27,201	9.4	9.2	9.4	−2.1
13	Essential (primary) hypertension and hypertensive renal disease	21,841	7.5	7.4	7.0	5.7
14	Parkinson's disease	17,898	6.2	6.1	5.9	3.4
15	Pneumonitis due to solids and liquids	17,457	6.0	5.9	6.1	−3.3
. . .	All other causes	421,226	144.8	. . .	. . .	. . .

—Quantity zero.
...Category not applicable.
*Rank based on number of deaths.

SOURCE: Donna L. Hoyert, Hsiang-Ching Kung, and Betty L. Smith, "Table B. Deaths and Death Rates for 2003 and Age-Adjusted Death Rates and Percent Changes in Age-Adjusted Rates from 2002 to 2003 for the 15 Leading Causes of Death in 2003: United States, Final 2002 and Preliminary 2003," in "Deaths: Preliminary Data for 2003," *National Vital Statistics Reports*, vol. 53, no. 15, Centers for Disease Control and Prevention, National Center for Health Statistics, February 28, 2005, http://www.cdc.gov/nchs/data/nvsr/nvsr53/nvsr53_15.pdf (accessed July 18, 2005)

FIGURE 1.1

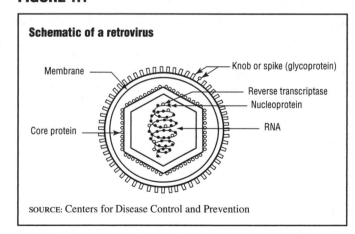

Schematic of a retrovirus

SOURCE: Centers for Disease Control and Prevention

African monkeys and in apes, with an infection rate ranging from 1 to 40%.

Max Essex and Phyllis T. Kanki of the Harvard School of Public Health in Boston, Massachusetts, discovered that the simian virus found in the African chimpanzee and the African green monkey was more homologous (related in primitive origin) to the human virus than to the simian virus in the Asian macaque. This discovery provided strong support for an evolved version of African STLV as being the origin of human HTLV.

In 1999 researchers from the University of Alabama announced their determination that the genetic sequence of a simian virus isolated from a tissue sample obtained from a chimpanzee was virtually identical to the HIV discovered by Montagnier. Interestingly, chimpanzees are only rarely infected with SIV. This implies that the chimpanzee may be a temporary "carrier" of the virus, which normally resides in some other, as yet unidentified, primate species.

The original HIV is now known as HIV-1. This is because of the 1986 discovery by scientists at the Pasteur Institute in Paris of a new AIDS-causing virus in West Africans. They labeled the virus HIV-2. The two forms of HIV have similar modes of transmission. But the symptoms of HIV-2 were found to be milder than those of HIV-1. Furthermore, HIV-2 was shown to differ in molecular structure from HIV-1 in a way that ties it more closely to a virus that causes AIDS in macaque monkeys. The CDC estimates that as of 1998, seventy-nine people in the United States had been infected with HIV-2. (Unless otherwise specified, the term "HIV" in the remainder of this publication refers to HIV-1.)

Along with the majority of investigators, Montagnier and Gallo believe that HIV has been present in Central Africa and other regions for some time. Presumably, at some point the virus crossed the species barrier from primates to humans. Currently, the most accepted theory is that this crossover resulted from a human eating meat from a chimpanzee or other primate. The rural nature of these societies and the limited access to the outside world by those infected with the virus may have confined the spread of HIV for many decades. But once migration of tribal Central Africans to urban areas began, the more liberated sexual practices there promoted the spread of HIV. Within a comparatively short time, the once rare and remote disease was spread by globe-trotting HIV-infected people.

Some other, more controversial theories propose that HIV was created in the laboratory, only to escape into the natural world. One theory is that the creation of one of the versions of the polio vaccine—which used primate tissue samples—was the source of the human infection. But examination of some of the original tissue samples stored at the Wistar Institute in Philadelphia in April 2001 failed to detect evidence of either HIV or SIV.

ATTACKING THE IMMUNE SYSTEM

As with other infections, HIV must evade the immune system, which functions to detect and destroy invaders. To learn how HIV first attacks healthy cells while evading attack by the immune system, it is important to understand the complex structure of HIV and how normal white blood cells work.

Healthy White Blood Cells at Work

White blood cells are major components of the complicated, coordinated system of organs and cells that make up the human immune system. These organs and cells work together to prevent invasion by foreign substances. There are five types of white blood cells: macrophages (scavenger cells of the immune system), T4 or helper T cells, T8 or killer T cells, plasma B cells, and memory B cells. T and B white blood cells are also called lymphocytes. It is these lymphocytes that bear the major responsibility for carrying out immune system activities.

Each type of white blood cell has a specific function. The macrophage, which begins as a smaller monocyte (single cell), readies the T4 cells to respond to particular invaders such as viruses. At the time of viral attack, the macrophage, sometimes referred to as the vacuum cleaner of the immune system, swallows the virus, but leaves a portion displayed so that the T4 cell can make contact. The macrophage also stimulates the production of thousands of T4 cells, which are all programmed to battle the invader.

When T4 lymphocytes attack an invading virus, they also send out chemical messages that cause the multiplication of B cells and T8 killer cells. These cells, along with the help of some T4 cells, destroy the infected cell.

Other T4 cells, which are not actively involved in destroying the infected cells, send chemical messages to B cells, causing them to reproduce and divide into groups of either plasma cells or memory cells. Plasma cells make antibodies that cripple the invading virus, while memory cells increase the immune response in the event that the invader ever attacks again.

HIV's Molecular Structure

HIV has nine genes. Three of these—designated env, gag, and pol code—form the structural components of the virus, such as the "coats" that surround the genetic material and form the outer surface of the virus particle. The remaining genes—tat, nef, rev, vpr, vpu, and vif—are involved in regulating the genetic activities that are necessary to create copies of the infecting virus.

HIV's compliment of nine genes is miniscule compared to the some thirty thousand genes that are in human DNA. Nevertheless, HIV is more complex than most other retroviruses, which have only three or four genes. Scientists believe that these genes direct the production of proteins that make up parts of the virus and regulate its reproduction. The HIV core contains genes that are protected by a protein shell, while the entire virus is surrounded by a fatty membrane dotted with glycoproteins (proteins with sugar units attached), adding to its protection. Figure 1.2, Figure 1.3, and Figure 1.4 show microscopic views of HIV in various stages of development.

Once HIV enters the human body, its primary target is a subset of immune cells that contain a molecule called CD4. In particular, the virus attaches itself to CD4+ T cells and, to a lesser extent, to macrophages.

A New Discovery

In 1995 researchers at Oxford University in England proposed that HIV defuses the killer cells that are supposed to destroy virus-stricken cells. The researchers isolated HIV from AIDS patients and demonstrated that the virus had undergone a mutation, or change, in its genetic structure. When killer T cells approached cells infected with the mutated virus, the T cells failed to kill the stricken cells, perhaps because they no longer recognized them. The T cells were in fact unable to kill even cells infected with the original, unmutated virus. The mutations not only allowed the altered strains to multiply, but also allowed unaltered strains to flourish.

ANOTHER THEORY: "FRIENDLY FIRE." Not all researchers agree that the alteration of killer T cells is the underlying basis for the establishment of an HIV infection. Some researchers believe instead that other cells in the immune system attack and kill CD4-containing cells in what has been termed an "autoimmune response." The CD4-containing cells that have not been invaded by

FIGURE 1.2

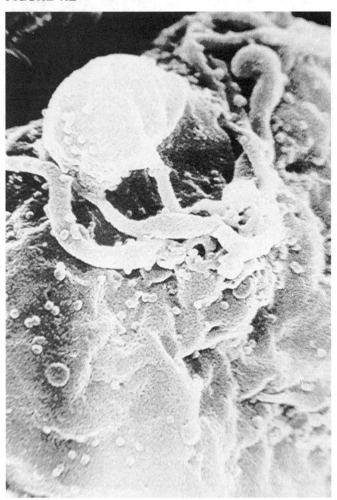

A scanning electron micrograph of HIV infected T4 lymphocytes, showing the virus budding from the plasma membrane of the lymphocytes. Centers for Disease Control and Prevention

FIGURE 1.4

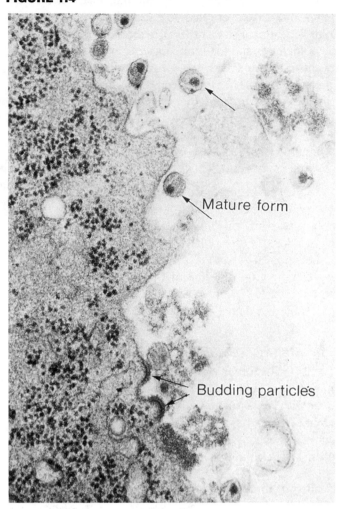

The HTLV-III/LAV-virus, found in a hemophilia patient who developed AIDS. Centers for Disease Control and Prevention

FIGURE 1.3

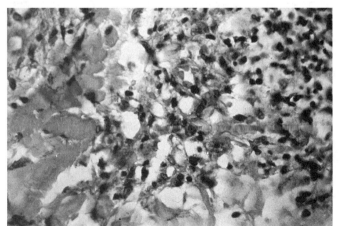

High magnification view of a T4 lymphocyte infected with HIV. Centers for Disease Control and Prevention

the virus, but display fragments of it, become targets for other cells—in addition to the killer cells—which see the infected cells as a camouflaged virus and kill them. In addition, HIV-infected cells may send out protein signals that weaken or destroy other healthy cells in the immune system.

Whatever the basis of the beginning of an HIV infection, it is agreed that HIV subsequently exhibits various behaviors, depending on the kind of cell it has invaded and how the cell behaves. The virus can remain dormant in T cells for two to twenty years, hidden from the immune system. When the cells are stimulated, however, the viral genes that have been incorporated into the DNA of the T4 cells can be replicated and the gene products assembled into new virus particles that then break free of the T4 cells and attack other cells. Once a T4 cell has been infected, it cannot respond adequately and may reproduce to form as few as ten cells. An uninfected T4 cell usually reproduces a thousand or more times to form the army needed to fight the HIV invader. When these crippled T4 cells do encounter the invader, the virus inside them reproduces and the cells are destroyed. To make the situation even worse, HIV reproduces itself at a rate far greater than any other known virus. The T4 cells essentially become factories for the invading enemy soldiers, ultimately producing them in overwhelming numbers.

The Attack

The immune system is unable to produce sufficient antibodies to fight off the complex HIV. The battle between HIV and the immune system begins when the virus slips into the bloodstream via a CD4 receptor enzyme on a T4 cell, to which it preferentially attaches itself. A CD4 receptor alone, however, is not enough to cause infection, and for years scientists searched for some other protein on the cell surface that HIV can exploit to gain entry.

This protein was discovered in May 1996 by a team of scientists at the National Institute of Allergy and Infectious Diseases (NIAID) in Bethesda, Maryland. The scientists named the protein "fusin" because it helps the virus fuse with a healthy cell membrane and inject genetic material into the cell. The CD4-containing cell signals to killer T cells that it is infected by displaying fragments of HIV proteins on its surface. This triggers the killer cells to spring into action, which multiply and seek out the infected CD4-containing cells in order to pierce them open and destroy them.

CONFIRMING A HIDING PLACE

Typically, an HIV infection begins with a sudden, flu-like illness. Shortly after this first episode, the virus virtually disappears and symptoms may not materialize for as long as twenty years. Over time, the immune system eventually collapses and the virus appears in ever-increasing amounts of CD4-containing cells floating free in the patient's blood. While previous studies focused on the presence of the virus in the blood, two independently conducted studies in 1993 confirmed suspicions long held by scientists that HIV hides in a patient's lymph nodes and similar tissue during the quiescent (first or early) stage of infection. In March 1993 Anthony S. Fauci et al. from NIAID and Ashley T. Haase et al. from the University of Minnesota published papers describing the hiding places of HIV (*Science*, Vol. 262, November 12, 1993).

Searching for an Active Virus

Research by Fauci and his colleagues focused on the search for the virus in the blood and lymphoid tissue (the lymph nodes, spleen, tonsils, and adenoids) of twelve HIV-infected patients whose infections had progressed to varying severities. Initially, the virus is concentrated almost entirely in the lymphoid tissues. Fauci et al. believe that the virus infiltrates the lymph nodes within weeks of the initial infection. Particles of the virus, coated with antibodies, adhere to the follicular dendritic cells, a group of filtering cells that trap foreign material. CD4-containing cells nearby "see" the trapped material and are stimulated to attack the invaders. The stronger virus counterattacks and reproduces itself on some of these CD4-containing cells.

After this infiltration, the performance of the immune system declines. This decline, which ultimately is dramatically debilitating, occurs over an extended period of time—up to twenty years in some AIDS sufferers. During this decline the follicular dendritic cells also begin to deteriorate, and the quantity of HIV in the CD4-containing cells floating free in the blood increases significantly. In the final stage of the disease there is an almost complete dissolution of the follicular dendritic cell network. At this point the amount of HIV in the blood and in the CD4-containing cells has grown to equal the amount in the lymph nodes.

NOT JUST THE IMMUNE SYSTEM

For some time scientists and researchers believed HIV attacked and affected only the immune system. Many early AIDS cases that provided evidence of the involvement of other regions of the body were not counted because of the narrower definitions of AIDS that existed before 1993. But after 1993 clear evidence showed that the free virus (not attached to any other cells) could appear in the fluid surrounding the brain and the spinal cord and in the bloodstream. HIV can be found not only in T4 lymphocytes but also in other immune system cells, as well as in cells in the nervous system, intestine, and bone marrow.

Researchers at the CDC proposed another reason why HIV infections are so difficult to eliminate and why the immune system appears to be so susceptible to them. Their research shows that HIV can infect and grow in very immature bone marrow cells, offering no clues about what the mature HIV-infected cells would become. The virus reproduces without revealing itself to the immune system, which under normal circumstances would destroy it. By developing in immature bone marrow cells, a great quantity of virus can be produced before the body ever attempts to resist it.

As they mature, the cells change, becoming infected monocytes and macrophages that may not only fail to fight infections, but may also spread the virus to other immune system cells. Infected marrow cells may seed the virus into other parts of the body, including the brain. The infected cells that develop in the marrow are carried through the bloodstream to the rest of the body.

SEARCHING FOR ANSWERS

Researchers have long been puzzled by the fact that AIDS is virtually always fatal, even though relatively small amounts of the virus are found in patients, compared to other lethal viral infections. How the virus acts to kill the cells has been hotly debated. Certainly, this behavior is inconsistent with other retroviruses, which do not kill all the infected host cells. Although HIV is considered a slow virus (a virus that exerts its effect over a long period of time), some AIDS activity occurs more quickly and may be associated with the coincidental presence of infectious mycoplasma (bacteria that lack a cell wall).

Restoring Immune Response

In December 1993 the NCI reported that the immune function had been restored to HIV-infected cells grown in a laboratory through the addition of interleukin-12 (IL-12). IL-12 is a member of a group of natural blood proteins called cytokines that were discovered in 1991 by scientists at the Wistar Institute in Philadelphia, Pennsylvania, and Hoffman-LaRoche Inc. in Nutley, New Jersey. Despite this promising result, the Food and Drug Administration (FDA) halted human testing of IL-12 in June 1995 when two patients died. After testing the protein on animals, researchers concluded that the problem was not in IL-12 itself, but in the timing of the doses. Consequently, human testing resumed in November 1995.

In December 1995 a new class of drugs called protease inhibitors received FDA approval. These drugs block the ability of HIV to mature and to infect new cells by suppressing the protein-degrading activity of a viral enzyme. Enzymes with this activity are classified as proteases, hence the designation of the enzyme blocker as a protease inhibitor. If protease inhibitors can block the spread of HIV in the immune system, then AIDS will not develop. Though patients may be HIV-positive the rest of their lives, they may never die from HIV infection.

Theories of HIV/AIDS Progression

Even after more than two decades of research, there is still no consensus among HIV experts as to the pathogenesis (the origination and development) of AIDS. Despite this, there is agreement that the latent period between the establishment of an HIV infection and the appearance of the symptoms of AIDS averages from about two to eleven years. But some people remain symptom-free for as long as twenty years. Furthermore, a select group of between 5 and 10% of all HIV-infected people does not appear to develop AIDS. Called "long-term nonprogressors," these individuals are believed to have genetic and immune response characteristics that slow, or may even halt, the course of disease progression. Much research interest centers on these people, since an

understanding of their physiological characteristics that allow them to suppress the infection could be invaluable to the treatment of the disease in other patients.

After HIV infection is established, the immune system regenerates cells only up to a certain point, which would explain a gradual progression to AIDS. The early regulatory functions of the immune system limit viral replication until a certain threshold is reached. When the number of different viral mutants becomes too large, the regulatory system is overwhelmed and shuts down, opening the door to opportunistic infections and eventual total decline.

When the total CD4+ T cell count falls from the normal 800 to 1,000 per cubic millimeter of blood to 200 per cubic millimeter, the rate of immune decline speeds up and the HIV-positive patient becomes prone to the opportunistic infections and other illnesses that are characteristic of AIDS. In searching for an antiretroviral therapy, researchers find that rather than boosting the CD4+ T cell count, interruption of the viral replication may be the way to reverse immune deficiency in HIV infection, though the nature of a reversing mechanism remains unknown.

SOME INCONSISTENCIES WITH CURRENT THEORIES. Most scientists agree that there are major gaps and inconsistencies in the knowledge of how HIV causes AIDS. One inconsistency deals with the infection and killing of the helper T cells. Initially, researchers thought that the main tactic of HIV was to infect and destroy the T cells. As these cells died, the numerical strength of the helper T cell force must be depleted, causing the immune deficiency associated with AIDS patients.

Other scientists, however, consider this theory too simplistic, since so few T cells—no more than one infected cell in 500—are infected. Rather, two studies published in 2001 in the *Journal of Experimental Medicine* (vol. 194) support the idea that HIV does not block the production of T cells but instead accelerates the division of existing T cells. This causes the existing T cells to die off more quickly than normal.

Another inconsistency involves the observation that the rapid decline in the number of T cells comes relatively late in the infection, even though there are clear indications that the immune system has been impaired much earlier.

NON-HIV THEORY OF AIDS: PETER DUESBERG. Finally, a theory championed by Peter Duesberg of the University of California, Berkeley, proposes that HIV is in fact not the cause of AIDS. Instead, Duesberg (*Journal of Bioscience*, vol. 28, no. 4, 2003) argues that AIDS in the United States "is a collection of chemical epidemics" resulting from the long-term consumption of recreational drugs, anti-HIV/AIDS drugs, and malnutrition. According

FIGURE 1.5

FIGURE 1.6

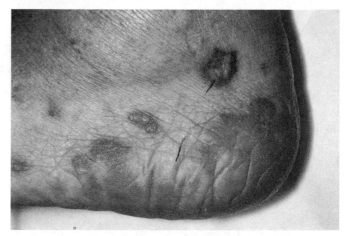

Violaceous plaques of Kaposi's sarcoma on the heel and lateral foot. Centers for Disease Control and Prevention

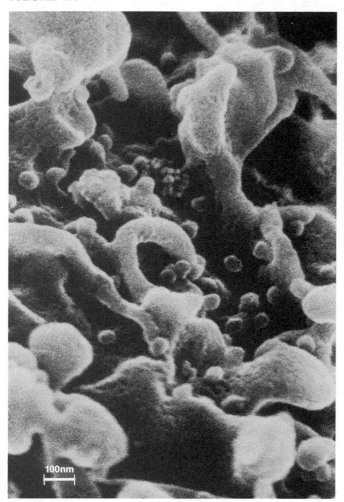

A skin biopsy of Kaposi's sarcoma. Centers for Disease Control and Prevention

to this hypothesis, AIDS is not contagious and HIV is a coincidental "passenger." This theory is extremely provocative and contentious and has not been accepted by the HIV/AIDS research community. Nonetheless, the theory does highlight some inconsistencies that have not been satisfactorily addressed to date.

CIGARETTES AND ALCOHOL SPEED DEVELOPMENT OF AIDS. Evidence that heavy cigarette smokers and chronic alcoholics can display a suppressed immune response has led some experts to believe that cigarette and alcohol use accelerates the development of AIDS symptoms. Accordingly, they counsel HIV-positive patients to abandon smoking and drinking alcohol.

OPPORTUNISTIC INFECTIONS

Once HIV has destroyed the immune system, the body can no longer protect itself against bacterial, fungal, protozoal, and other viral agents that take advantage of the compromised condition and cause infections. These infections, which would not otherwise occur but for an impaired immune system, are known as opportunistic infections (OIs). In the non-AIDS community, OIs are problematic in hospitals, where ill, newborn, or elderly patients also display a less than adequately functioning immune system. Because the patient is considered to have AIDS if at least one OI appears, OIs are also referred to as "AIDS-defining events," though OIs are not the only AIDS-defining events.

By 1997 the leading OI for Americans suffering from HIV/AIDS was *Pneumocystis carinii* pneumonia (PCP), a lung disease caused by a fungus. This dominance has continued through 2005. Prior to the discovery of HIV/AIDS, PCP was found almost exclusively in cancer and transplant patients with weakened immune systems. PCP has been declining since 1987, most likely due to better treatment and earlier diagnosis. Esophageal candidiasis, an infection of the esophagus, and extrapulmonary cryptococcosis, a systemic fungus that enters the body through the lungs and may invade any organ of the body, are also OIs frequently diagnosed in AIDS patients.

Other illnesses such as Burkitt's lymphoma, invasive cervical cancer, and primary brain lymphoma are also considered AIDS-defining events. Wasting syndrome (which includes sudden weight loss and lethargy) is another illness that may be considered an AIDS-defining event. Other examples of AIDS-defining events include diagnosis of *Mycobacterium avium* complex (MAC), a serious bacterial infection that may occur in one part of the body such as the liver, bone marrow, and spleen or spread throughout the body; cytomegalovirus disease, a member of the herpesvirus group; Kaposi's sarcoma, a once-rare cancer of the blood vessel walls that causes conspicuous purple lesions on the skin (see Figure 1.5 and Figure 1.6); and toxoplasmic encephalitis, an inflammation of the brain. Patients may experience more than one OI or AIDS-defining event.

HIV and Tuberculosis

Tuberculosis (TB) is a communicable infection caused by the bacterium *Mycobacterium tuberculosis*. TB was a widespread epidemic in North America in the late nineteenth and early twentieth centuries. Subsequently, it faded from prominence. But TB regained a foothold in the 1990s, with the number of cases increasing in the United States. Part of this increase is the parallel increase in the occurrence of the infection in HIV-positive individuals. Indeed, HIV infection has become one of the strongest known risk factors for the progression of TB from infection to disease.

An important 1996 report from the Conference on Retroviruses and Opportunistic Infections first concluded that the decline in CD4+ T cells is greater in HIV-infected patients who develop TB than in those who remain free of TB. In some geographic areas up to 58% of those diagnosed with TB were also HIV-positive. Of the many diseases associated with HIV infection, TB is one of the few that is transmissible, treatable, and preventable.

TB is spread from person to person through the inhalation of airborne particles containing *M. tuberculosis*. The particles, called droplet nuclei, are produced when a person with infectious TB of the lung or larynx forcefully exhales, such as when coughing, sneezing, speaking, or singing. These infectious particles remain suspended in the air and may be inhaled by someone sharing the same air. Risk of transmission is increased where ventilation is poor and when susceptible people share air for prolonged periods with a person who has untreated pulmonary TB.

Approximately 85% of TB infections occur in the lungs. This infection is termed "pulmonary TB." But TB may occur at any site of the body, such as the larynx, the lymph nodes, the brain, the kidneys, or the bones. These cases are termed extrapulmonary TB. With the exception of laryngeal TB, people with extrapulmonary TB are usually not considered infectious to others. It is important to note that, as mentioned earlier in this chapter, HIV is a blood-borne infection and cannot be spread through air. An HIV-positive person who has TB can spread TB nuclei through the air, but not HIV.

TB does not develop in everyone who is infected with the bacteria. In the United States about 90% of the infections are lifelong, yet those infected never develop symptoms of TB. But in about 5% of people, the disease develops in the first or second year after infection, and in another 5% it develops later in life. The risk that TB symptoms will develop in people with both TB and HIV is about 8% per year. In contrast, the risk that TB will develop in those infected only with *M. tuberculosis* is 5 to 10% within their lifetime.

HIV and Cancer

People with AIDS are susceptible to cancer. Some malignant tumors, such as Kaposi's sarcoma and cancers of the lymph system, have been common among AIDS patients since the disease was first discovered in 1981. More recently, however, physicians and researchers are beginning to find that certain forms of cancer are becoming prevalent among HIV/AIDS patients who are living longer.

Most AIDS-related cancers are believed to be caused by viruses. These cancers are more common among HIV-infected people because HIV suppresses the immune system, enabling cancer-causing viruses to attack more successfully. These cancers include non-Hodgkin's lymphoma (found in lymph tissues) and primary lymphoma of the brain. People infected with HIV are also at greater risk of myeloma (malignant tumors of the bone marrow), brain tumors, testicular cancers, and leukemia.

Since newer anti-HIV combination drug therapies, such as highly active antiretroviral therapy (HAART), have become available, researchers have reported a decline in Kaposi's sarcoma and primary lymphoma of the brain. One possible explanation for the decline may be that the combination drug therapies enable the body to recover partial immunity, which in turn controls the cancer. While the decline appears real, investigators believe it is too early to accept these findings until a longer-term follow-up has been completed.

TOWARD A VACCINE: THE HOPE AND THE REALITIES

The different routes of attack of HIV on the immune system and the ability of the virus to mutate has prompted the suggestion by some researchers that the development of an effective vaccine will be difficult to achieve. This admission is very different from the day in 1984 when Margaret Heckler, the secretary of the Department of Health and Human Services under President Ronald Reagan, announced that the identification of HIV would lead to a vaccine within two years.

The intervening years have made many AIDS researchers realize that the chances of developing a vaccine that would prevent AIDS (confer immunity on the person receiving the vaccine) are remote. Testing the effectiveness of an AIDS vaccine is also difficult, since the deliberate contamination of people with HIV is both unethical and illegal. The focus of research has shifted to vaccines that do not prevent infections but rather lessen their effects and delay the progress of the disease.

Such vaccine efforts continue. At the end of 2001 NIAID and the international HIV Vaccine Trials Network announced an agreement with Merck & Co., a leading manufacturer of anti-HIV compounds, to support the evaluation of promising HIV vaccines. The agreement with Merck was expected to spur evaluation of still more candidate vaccines. According to the HIV Vaccine Trials Network, as of May 2005 sixteen vaccine trials are underway on 3,639 enrolled participants.

In the mid-1990s a "hit-hard-early" strategy gained favor. In this strategy a cocktail of anti-HIV drugs was given to patients soon after diagnosis of the presence of the virus. The idea of HAART is to suppress the reproduction of the virus as much as possible. HAART shows promise. Some of the drugs target the virus's reverse transcriptase. By inhibiting the enzyme's activity, the ability of HIV to reproduce is thwarted. But HAART has a downside. The therapy is expensive and hard to maintain, and its long-term use is associated with a number of serious side effects. A "seven-day-on, seven-day-off" pattern of HAART (structured treatment interruptions) produces promising results. While it is still too early to say whether these structured interruptions will be incorporated into the normal course of therapy, it is conceivable that, in the future, the side effects of HAART may be lessened by the use of intermittent therapy.

CHAPTER 2

DEFINITION, SYMPTOMS, AND TRANSMITTAL

A DEFINITION OF AIDS

The Centers for Disease Control and Prevention (CDC) in Atlanta, Georgia, a branch of the U.S. Public Health Service, is the federal government's clearinghouse, research center, and monitoring agency for all infectious diseases, including HIV/AIDS. The CDC tracks the diseases in the United States and notifies health officials of their occurrence via *Morbidity and Mortality Weekly Report* notices and a Web site that is updated frequently.

The CDC defines AIDS as a specific group of diseases or conditions that are indicative of severe immunosuppression related to infection with HIV. The health agency first outlined a surveillance (a constant observation of a process) case definition in 1982, then revised it in 1983, 1985, 1987, 1993, and again in 2000 as knowledge about HIV infection increased and additional severe and common symptoms were included in the definitions. The January 1, 1993, definition emphasized the clinical importance of the CD4+ T cell count and included the addition of three clinical conditions.

THE 1993 CLASSIFICATION REVISION AND EXPANDED SURVEILLANCE CASE DEFINITION

In 1991 the CDC released a draft of the document that would become the *1993 Revised Classification for HIV Infection and Expanded AIDS Surveillance Case Definition for Adolescents and Adults*. This classification scheme has not been revised in the intervening years and so remains the standard in 2005.

The revision addressed the concerns of many women, their attorneys, and physicians, who had strongly advocated the inclusion of diseases such as pelvic inflammatory disease and vaginal candidiasis as conditions that could precede the development of AIDS, so that women infected with HIV would be included in the revised definition. Advocates cautioned that if the CDC omitted such inclusive criteria, many women would be denied access to disability benefits, necessary treatment, and education.

Reasons for Expanding the Case Definition

The CDC reported three reasons for expanding the AIDS surveillance case definitions:

1. **To be consistent with standards of medical care for HIV-infected people**. The addition of a measurement for severe immunosuppression—a CD4+ T lymphocyte count of 200 per cubic millimeter or less than 14% of total lymphocytes—is consistent with the standard used to determine clinical and therapeutic treatment of HIV-infected persons. (It is important to note that a person can be HIV infected and not have AIDS.) Some clinicians recommend a conservative approach, that all persons with a count of 500 CD4+ T cells per cubic millimeter or less be given antiretroviral therapy. Others advocate more aggressive treatment and begin antiretroviral therapy as soon as the diagnosis of HIV infection is made. Prophylaxis (prevention treatment) against *Pneumocystis carinii* pneumonia (PCP), the most common serious opportunistic infection (OI), should be started on patients with a count of 200 CD4+ T cells per cubic millimeter or less.

2. **To include people with conditions of major public health importance in the HIV epidemic**. The inclusion of HIV-infected people with low CD4+ T cell counts allows the HIV/AIDS surveillance to reflect more accurately the number of people who have severe immunosuppression. These people are in the greatest need of close medical follow-up and are at the greatest risk for many or all of the severe HIV-related illnesses. The addition of three clinical conditions—pulmonary tuberculosis (TB), recurrent pneumonia, and invasive cervical cancer—to the

twenty-three already accepted conditions of AIDS surveillance criteria indicates the documented or potential importance of these diseases in the HIV epidemic. The prognoses for both pulmonary TB and cervical cancer are improved with appropriate screening tests and proper follow-up. The third condition, recurrent pneumonia, was included to show the importance of pulmonary infections in the causes of HIV-related diseases and deaths.

3. **To simplify the AIDS case-reporting process.** The CDC tried to simplify the AIDS case-reporting process by allowing clinicians to report HIV-infected people on the basis of CD4+ T cell counts. Limited staff at outpatient clinics and the increasing proportion of AIDS cases necessitated the use of a simplified AIDS surveillance case definition.

New Definition and Classification—Tied to CD4+ Cells

One of the major obstacles in defining AIDS has been that it is not a single disease but several diseases making up a syndrome (a syndrome is a group or pattern of symptoms or abnormalities that are indicative of a certain disease). Newer preventive treatments delay the onset of many diseases such as PCP, which in the past helped to define AIDS. In order to obtain a more realistic picture of the number of AIDS cases, the new classification system emphasized the importance of the CD4+ or helper T cell count.

Based on this, the 1993 definition included all HIV-infected people with a CD4+ T cell count of less than 200 per cubic millimeter or whose CD4+ T cell count was less than 14% of total lymphocytes. Essentially, most people with very low T4 counts would be defined as having AIDS. As shown in Table 2.1, the 1993 classification system was based on three ranges of CD4+ T cell counts (1, 2, 3) and three clinical categories (A, B, C), with nine combinations being possible (A1, A2, A3, B1, B2, B3, C1, C2, C3). People with AIDS-indicator conditions (category C) or those with CD4+ T cell counts of less than 200 per cubic millimeter meet the immunologic criteria for the AIDS surveillance case definition.

Table 2.2 gives a more detailed description of categories A and B, as well as the clinical conditions listed in category C. Note that for classification purposes, once a category C (AIDS indicator) condition occurred, the person remained in category C.

The Impact of the 1993 Definition on Case Reporting

CDC data indicates that expansion of the AIDS surveillance criteria changed both the process of AIDS surveillance and the number of reported cases. During 1993, local, state, and territorial health departments reported 103,500 AIDS cases in the United States among adults and adolescents thirteen years of age and older.

TABLE 2.1

Classification system for HIV infection and expanded surveillance case definition for AIDS among adolescents and adults[a]

CD4+ T-cell categories	Clinical categories		
	(A) Asymptomatic, acute (primary) HIV or PGL[b]	(B) Symptomatic, not (A) or (C) conditions	(C) AIDS-indicator conditions
(1) ≥500/μL	A1	B1	C1
(2) 200–499/μL	A2	B2	C2
(3) <200/μL AIDS-indicator T-cell count	A3	B3	C3

[a]The shaded cells illustrate the expanded AIDS surveillance case definition. Persons with AIDS-indicator conditions (category C) as well as those with CD4+ T-lymphocyte counts <200/μL (categories A3 or B3) will be reportable as AIDS cases in the United States and territories, effective January 1, 1993.
[b]PGL=persistent generalized lymphadenopathy. Clinical category A includes acute (primary) HIV infection.

SOURCE: "1993 Revised Classification System for HIV Infection and Expanded Surveillance Case Definition for AIDS among Adolescents and Adults," in *Morbidity and Mortality Weekly Report*, vol. 41, no. RR-17, Centers for Disease Control and Prevention, December 18, 1992, http://www.cdc.gov/mmwr/preview/mmwrhtml/00018871.htm (accessed July 18, 2005)

This number was twice the 49,016 cases reported in 1992 and likely represented a one-time effect of the 1993 expansion of the AIDS definition. (See Figure 2.1.) The steep increase probably represented the reporting of people who were diagnosed with the newly added conditions before 1993. New reported AIDS cases declined again beginning in 1996 in response to treatments, such as highly active antiretroviral therapy (HAART), that slowed the progression from HIV infection to AIDS. During 1998–1999 the decline in the incidence of AIDS began to level. From 1999 to 2001 essentially no change (or a very slight increase) occurred. But from 2001 through 2003 the number of reported cases again rose, albeit modestly. (See Figure 2.1.)

THE 2000 REVISED SURVEILLANCE CASE DEFINITION

On December 10, 1999, the CDC released a revised surveillance case definition, updating the definition for HIV infection implemented in 1993. (See Table 2.3.) Effective January 1, 2000, the revision integrated the reporting for adult and pediatric HIV infection and AIDS into a single-case definition. The new definition was based on new data obtained using the more sensitive and specific HIV diagnostic tests that were not yet available at the time of the 1993 revision of the AIDS definition. These newer tests detect HIV DNA or RNA; the earlier tests only detected anti-HIV antibodies. The newer tests allow for HIV detection in nearly all infants age one month or older. Since newborns might not have expressed anti-HIV antibodies—if their immune systems have even matured enough to be capable of antibody expression—they would be negative using an antibody-based test.

TABLE 2.2

Clinical categories of AIDS infection

Category A

Category A consists of one or more of the conditions listed below in an adolescent or adult (≥13 years) with documented HIV infection. Conditions listed in Categories B and C must not have occurred.

- Asymptomatic HIV infection
- Persistent generalized lymphadenopathy
- Acute (primary) HIV infection with accompanying illness or history of acute HIV infection

Category B

Category B consists of symptomatic conditions in an HIV-infected adolescent or adult that are not included among conditions listed in clinical Category C and that meet at least one of the following criteria: a) the conditions are attributed to HIV infection or are indicative of a defect in cell-mediated immunity; or b) the conditions are considered by physicians to have a clinical course or to require management that is complicated by HIV infection. Examples of conditions in clinical Category B include, but are not limited to:

- Bacillary angiomatosis
- Candidiasis, oropharyngeal (thrush)
- Candidiasis, vulvovaginal; persistent, frequent, or poorly responsive to therapy
- Cervical dysplasia/moderate or severe cervical carcinoma in situ
- Constitutional symptoms, such as fever (38.5° C) or diarrhea lasting >1 month
- Hairy leukoplakia, oral
- Herpes zoster (shingles), involving at least two distinct episodes or more than one dermatome
- Idiopathic thrombocytopenic purpura
- Listeriosis
- Pelvic inflammatory disease, particularly if complicated by tubo-ovarian abscess
- Peripheral neuropathy

For classification purposes, Category B conditions take precedence over those in Category A. For example, someone previously treated for oral or persistent vaginal candidiasis (and who has not developed a Category C disease) but who is now asymptomatic should be classified in clinical Category B.

Category C

Category C includes the clinical conditions listed in the AIDS surveillance case definition. For classification purposes, once a Category C condition has occurred, the person will remain in Category C.

Conditions included in the 1993 AIDS surveillance case definition

- Candidiasis of bronchi, trachea, or lungs
- Candidiasis, esophageal
- Cervical cancer, invasive*
- Coccidioidomycosis, disseminated or extrapulmonary
- Cryptococcosis, extrapulmonary
- Cryptosporidiosis, chronic intestinal (>1 month's duration)
- Cytomegalovirus disease (other than liver, spleen, or nodes)
- Cytomegalovirus retinitis (with loss of vision)
- Encephalopathy, HIV-related
- Herpes simplex: chronic ulcer(s) (>1 month's duration); or bronchitis, pneumonitis, or esophagitis
- Histoplasmosis, disseminated or extrapulmonary
- Isosporiasis, chronic intestinal (>1 month's duration)
- Kaposi's sarcoma
- Lymphoma, Burkitt's (or equivalent term)
- Lymphoma, immunoblastic (or equivalent term)
- Lymphoma, primary, of brain
- *Mycobacterium avium* complex *or M. kansasii,* disseminated or extrapulmonary
- *Mycobacterium tuberculosis, any site* (pulmonary* or extrapulmonary)
- *Mycobacterium,* other species or unidentified species, disseminated or extrapulmonary
- *Pneumocystis carinii* pneumonia
- Pneumonia, recurrent*
- Progressive multifocal leukoencephalopathy
- *Salmonella* septicemia, recurrent
- Toxoplasmosis of brain
- Wasting syndrome due to HIV

*Added in the 1993 expansion of the AIDS surveillance case definition.

SOURCE: "1993 Revised Classification System for HIV Infection and Expanded Surveillance Case Definition for AIDS among Adolescents and Adults," in *Morbidity and Mortality Weekly Report*, vol. 41, no. RR-17, Centers for Disease Control and Prevention, December 18, 1992

Although reporting criteria include recommendations for diagnosing HIV infection, the primary purpose of the original and updated case definitions for HIV and AIDS is public health surveillance as opposed to the diagnosis of individual patients.

DIAGNOSIS AND SYMPTOMS OF AIDS

Only a qualified health professional can diagnose AIDS. To evaluate a patient with a positive HIV test, the health care practitioner performs a complete physical examination and collects the patient's social and family history. Diagnostic laboratory tests are also performed. These tests typically include complete blood count and routine chemistry; CD4+ T cell count; assays (analyses) that measure the amount of HIV-1 RNA in plasma; tuberculin skin tests to detect the presence of the bacterium that causes tuberculosis; and assays for the microbial agents that cause syphilis, toxoplasmosis, and hepatitis B

FIGURE 2.1

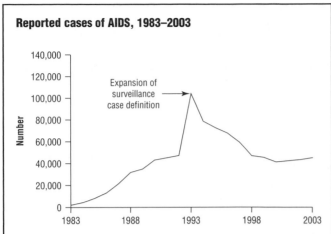

Reported cases of AIDS, 1983–2003

During 1994–2000, the number of AIDS cases reported to CDC decreased 47.4%, predominantly attributable to effective antiretroviral therapies. During 2000–2003, the number of reported AIDS cases increased 8.5%. This increase might be attributable to increased AIDS case ascertainment in areas with recent HIV reporting implementation.

SOURCE: "Acquired Immunodeficiency Syndrome (AIDS). Number of Reported Cases, by Year—United States and U.S. Territories, 1983–2003," in "Summary of Notifiable Diseases—United States, 2003," *Morbidity and Mortality Weekly Report*, vol. 53, no. 54, Centers for Disease Control and Prevention, April 22, 2005, http://www.cdc.gov/mmwr/preview/mmwrhtml/mm5254a1.htm (accessed July 18, 2005)

and C. Female patients are screened for cervical cancer using the cervical *Papanicolaou* ("pap") smear.

HIV infection progresses through a range of stages. Following the establishment of the infection (primary infection) there follows a typically prolonged asymptomatic (symptom-free) period prior to the appearance of symptoms and the deterioration of the patient's health. Among the symptoms that develop are weight loss; malaise; nausea; fever; night sweats; swollen lymph glands; a heavy, persistent, dry cough; easy bruising or unexplained bleeding; watery diarrhea; loss of memory; balance problems; mood changes; blurring or loss of vision; and oral lesions, such as thrush (a fungal infection caused by *Candida albicans*, which appears as a white coating of the tongue and throat). The infecting virus is basically the same in all infected people in terms of its structure and genetic makeup, but individual reactions to the virus vary greatly. Death is usually the result of the OIs and cancers that arise due to the impaired immune system—not HIV.

Dementia

Prior to the *1987 Case Definition* many researchers were reluctant to include dementia as a symptom indicative of AIDS. Some observers cited early studies that showed as many as 40 to 70% of people infected with the virus developed neurological and psychological complications several years before other clinical symptoms, such as weight loss and fever, appeared. This fear led

both military and civilian authorities to bar infected people from certain jobs involving public safety, including commercial pilots and bus drivers.

Officials at the World Health Organization (WHO), headquartered in Geneva, Switzerland, and the National Institutes of Health (NIH) in Bethesda, Maryland, jointly found these estimates to be false. They reported that although neurological complications are common in the later stages of AIDS, dementia is rarely diagnosed in asymptomatic HIV-infected persons, affecting fewer than 1% of those infected with HIV who have not yet developed AIDS.

A number of research studies were initiated in the 1990s to determine conclusively the link (if any) between dementia and the subsequent diagnosis of AIDS. The data from studies conducted by the U.S. Air Force, a joint effort by the CDC and the San Francisco Health Department, and the Multicenter AIDS Cohort Study of men who have sex with other men in Baltimore, Chicago, Los Angeles, and Pittsburgh (sponsored by the National Institute of Allergy and Infectious Diseases and the National Cancer Institute) confirmed that the 40 to 70% frequency rate of dementia for HIV-infected people was far higher than the actual rate. One explanation for the higher figures reported into the 1980s is that the data came from centers to which AIDS patients with dementia had been referred for treatment. Put another way, the sample population was skewed toward the increased prevalence of dementia.

HIV-associated dementia (also called AIDS dementia complex) is now recognized as a declining cognitive (thinking) function that generally occurs in the late stages of HIV infection. The dementia is caused directly by the destruction of brain cells by the infecting HIV and is different from the forgetfulness and difficulty in concentrating that can be by-products of depression and fatigue.

From HIV to AIDS

Through 2004 the average amount of time from the initial HIV infection to the development of AIDS was eleven years. Still, some patients are HIV-positive for up to twenty years before developing AIDS. The survival time after an AIDS diagnosis has markedly increased since the 1980s. More than two decades ago, death normally followed within two years of diagnosis. But medical developments during the 1980s and 1990s, such as the use of HAART, have significantly increased the life expectancy of AIDS patients.

THE EARLY STAGE. While the timing and progression of HIV infection vary among people, the disease follows a basic pattern. In the beginning of the early stage, shortly after the virus has entered the bloodstream, the T4 cell count is normal (around 1,000 per cubic milli-

TABLE 2.3

Revised surveillance case definition for HIV infection[a]

This revised definition of HIV infection, which applies to any HIV (e.g., HIV-1 or HIV-2), is intended for public health surveillance only. It incorporates the reporting criteria for HIV infection and AIDS into a single case definition. The revised criteria for HIV infection update the definition of HIV infection implemented in 1993; the revised HIV criteria apply to AIDS-defining conditions for adults and children, which require laboratory evidence of HIV. This definition is **not** presented as a guide to clinical diagnosis or for other uses.

I. **In adults, adolescents, or children aged ≥18 months[b], a reportable case of HIV infection must meet at least one of the following criteria:**

Laboratory criteria

Positive result on a screening test for HIV antibody (e.g., repeatedly reactive enzyme immunoassay), followed by a positive result on a confirmatory (sensitive and more specific) test for HIV antibody (e.g., Western blot or immunofluorescence antibody test)

or

Positive result or report of a detectable quantity on any of the following HIV virologic (nonantibody) tests:

- HIV nucleic acid (DNA or RNA) detection (e.g., DNA polymerase chain reaction [PCR] or plasma HIV-1 RNA)[c]
- HIV p24 antigen test, including neutralization assay
- HIV isolation (viral culture)

OR

Clinical or other criteria (if the above laboratory criteria are not met)

Diagnosis of HIV infection, based on the laboratory criteria above, that is documented in a medical record by a physician

or

Conditions that meet criteria included in the case definition for AIDS

II. **In a child aged <18 months, a reportable case of HIV infection must meet at least one of the following criteria:**

Laboratory criteria

Definitive

Positive results on two separate specimens (excluding cord blood) using one or more of the following HIV virologic (nonantibody) tests:

- HIV nucleic acid (DNA or RNA) detection
- HIV p24 antigen test, including neutralization assay, in a child ≥1 month of age
- HIV isolation (viral culture)

or

Presumptive

A child who does not meet the criteria for definitive HIV infection but who has:

Positive results on only one specimen (excluding cord blood) using the above HIV virologic tests and no subsequent negative HIV virologic or negative HIV antibody tests

OR

Clinical or other criteria (if the above definitive or presumptive laboratory criteria are not met)

Diagnosis of HIV infection, based on the laboratory criteria above, that is documented in a medical record by a physician

or

Conditions that meet criteria included in the 1987 pediatric surveillance case definition for AIDS

meter). The virus is undetectable at this stage using assays that are geared to detect the presence of anti-HIV antibodies. The antibody assays can remain negative for up to six weeks. In unusual cases antibodies may remain undetectable for a year or more. Even after testing positive for the virus, or for the presence of the antiviral antibodies, many people remain asymptomatic (showing no symptoms) for years. These people may develop a disorder similar to infectious mononucleosis with fatigue, fever, swollen glands, and possibly a rash. Often, these symptoms disappear within a few weeks and a connection with HIV infection is not made. Throughout this time, however, the virus is multiplying and destroying healthy cells. Most people continue to feel fine, though some may have chronically swollen lymph nodes. This stage usually lasts about five years.

THE MIDDLE STAGE. By the middle stage of infection, the CD4+ T cell count is reduced by half, to around 500 per cubic millimeter. Even with this physiological change, many people may still be asymptomatic. As the infection advances, skin tests will likely show that cell-mediated immunity, a form of immunological defense, is disintegrating. The deterioration of the immune system has begun. This stage can also last up to five years.

In the 1980s a drug called azidothymidine (AZT; now also called zidovudine), which had failed to fulfill its early potential as an anticancer compound, garnered a lot of publicity when it was shown to help slow the attachment of HIV to host cells. AZT delayed the onset of symptoms and extended this middle stage of the infection. Disappointingly, AZT's benefits proved to be temporary, as HIV mutated to counteract the effect of the drug. The drug is still used today in conjunction with other medicines, and some studies suggest that people who receive AZT may develop AIDS later than those who do not take it.

Newer and more promising drugs have since been developed, in particular the protease inhibitors, which prevent the virus from destructively degrading cell protein. Protease inhibitors were licensed for use by the U.S. Food and Drug Administration (FDA) in December 1995.

Structured treatment interruptions (STIs), initially proposed in the late 1990s, in which the multiple drug

TABLE 2.3

Revised surveillance case definition for HIV infection[a] [CONTINUED]

III. A child aged <18 months born to an HIV-infected mother will be categorized for surveillance purposes as "not infected with HIV" if the child does not meet the criteria for HIV infection but meets the following criteria:

Laboratory criteria

Definitive

At least two negative HIV antibody tests from separate specimens obtained at ≥6 months of age

or

At least two negative HIV virologic tests[4] from separate specimens, both of which were performed at ≥1 month of age and one of which was performed at ≥4 months of age

AND

No other laboratory or clinical evidence of HIV infection (i.e., has not had any positive virologic tests, if performed, and has not had an AIDS-defining condition)

or

Presumptive

A child who does not meet the above criteria for definitive "not infected" status but who has:

One negative EIA HIV antibody test performed at ≥6 months of age and NO positive HIV virologic tests, if performed

or

One negative HIV virologic test[d] performed at ≥4 months of age and NO positive HIV virologic tests, if performed

or

One positive HIV virologic test with at least two subsequent negative virologic tests[4], at least one of which is at ≥4 months of age; or negative HIV antibody test results, at least one of which is at ≥6 months of age

AND

No other laboratory or clinical evidence of HIV infection (i.e., has not had any positive virologic tests, if performed, and has not had an AIDS-defining condition).

OR

Clinical or other criteria (if the above definitive or presumptive laboratory criteria are not met)

Determined by a physician to be "not infected", and a physician has noted the results of the preceding HIV diagnostic tests in the medical record

AND

NO other laboratory or clinical evidence of HIV infection (i.e., has not had any positive virologic tests, if performed, and has not had an AIDS-defining condition)

IV. A child aged <18 months born to an HIV-infected mother will be categorized as having perinatal exposure to HIV infection if the child does not meet the criteria for HIV infection (II) or the criteria for "not infected with HIV" (III).

[a]Draft revised surveillance criteria for HIV infection were approved and recommended by the membership of the Council of State and Territorial Epidemiologists (CSTE) at the 1998 annual meeting. Draft versions of these criteria were previously reviewed by state HIV/AIDS surveillance staffs, CDC, CSTE, and laboratory experts. In addition, the pediatric criteria were reviewed by an expert panel of consultants. [External Pediatric Consultants: C. Hanson, M. Kaiser, S. Paul, G. Scott, and P. Thomas. CDC staff: J. Bertolli, K. Dominguez, M. Kalish, M.L. Lindegren, M. Rogers, C. Schable, R.J. Simonds, and J. Ward]
[b]Children aged ≥18 months but <13 years are categorized as "not infected with HIV" if they meet the criteria in III.
[c]In adults, adolescents, and children infected by other than perinatal exposure, plasma viral RNA nucleic acid tests should **NOT** be used in lieu of licensed HIV screening tests (e.g., repeatedly reactive enzyme immunoassay). In addition, a negative (i.e., undetectable) plasma HIV-1 RNA test result does not rule out the diagnosis of HIV infection.
[d]HIV nucleic acid (DNA or RNA) detection tests are the virologic methods of choice to exclude infection in children aged <18 months. Although HIV culture can be used for this purpose, it is more complex and expensive to perform and is less well standardized than nucleic acid detection tests. The use of p24 antigen testing to exclude infection in children aged <18 months is not recommended because of its lack of sensitivity.

SOURCE: "Revised Surveillance Case Definition for HIV Infection," in "CDC Guidelines for National Immunodeficiency Virus Case Surveillance Including Monitoring for HIV and AIDS," *Morbidity and Mortality Weekly Report*, vol. 48, no. RR-13, Centers for Disease Control and Prevention, December 10, 1999

---

therapy patients receive is stopped for short periods of time, have also shown promise. But the disastrous consequences that have resulted from patients taking self-initiated "drug holidays" underscore the importance of gaining a physician's approval for being on an STI program. As of 2005 it remains unclear whether STI truly does help suppress or delay AIDS symptoms.

THE LATE STAGE. The third and final stage of HIV infection is reached when the CD4+ T cell count per cubic millimeter drops to 200 or below. Though many patients are still asymptomatic at this point, the functioning of the immune system has by now been markedly weakened. The body is far less able to defend itself from invasion. As a consequence, the risk of infection due to opportunistic bacteria, viruses, fungi, and parasites and the possibility of cancer increase dramatically. In order to prevent PCP, one of the most common OIs,

patients are usually treated with antibiotics during this stage.

At the onset of the late stage, patients may experience weight loss, diarrhea, lethargy, and recurring fever. Skin and mucous membrane infections increase. Oral fungal infections such as thrush and a chronic infection caused by the herpes simplex virus are common.

As the late stage progresses, the immune system begins to collapse rapidly. OIs move deeper into the body. It is not uncommon for a parasitic infection called toxoplasmosis to attack the brain, while the cryptococcosis fungus attacks the nervous system, liver, bones, and skin. Cytomegalovirus can cause pneumonia, encephalitis, and retinitis. The latter, an inflammation of the retina, can cause blindness. Many other infections can occur. The consequences and complications of compromised immune function are numerous, and death becomes a matter of time. The average survival rate, once the late stage has been reached, is two years.

TRANSMISSION OF HIV

When AIDS was first discovered, it was often compared to the Black Death of the fourteenth century, in terms of the public panic surrounding the disease and its possible spread. The comparison has not proved to be valid. The bacterium that caused the Black Death (and which still causes bubonic plague) is very contagious, being readily transmitted via food, water, and air. HIV is not nearly as contagious. Moreover, by observing precautions that prevent the sharing of bodily fluids, the transmission of HIV can be almost entirely prevented.

The accumulated knowledge of more than twenty years of research and observations have definitively established that the HIV infection can only be transmitted by the following routes:

- Oral, anal, or vaginal sex with an infected person. Sexual intercourse—particularly heterosexual sex— is the most common mode of HIV transmission.

- Sharing drug needles or syringes with an infected person.

- Maternal transmission to a baby perinatally (at the time of birth) and possibly through breast milk.

- Transplantation of HIV-infected organs or transfusion of infected bodily fluids, such as blood or blood products. In the mid-1980s the transfusion of HIV-infected blood caused thousands of cases of AIDS and led to many deaths in separate incidents in Europe, the United States, and Canada. The blood agencies of the affected countries have revamped their blood-testing policies so that molecular assay techniques, which detect HIV genetic material, are used to screen every donated blood sample.

Confirming the involvement of bodily fluids in HIV transmission, high concentrations of HIV have been found in blood, semen, and cerebrospinal fluid. Not all body fluids seem to be involved, since HIV concentrations one thousand times less have been found in saliva, tears, vaginal secretions, breast milk, and feces. But there have been no reports of HIV transmission from saliva, tears, or human bites. In fact, in 1995 the National Institute of Dental Research in Bethesda, Maryland, reported that a small protein found in human saliva actually blocks the virus from entering the system.

Casual Contact

While HIV is an infectious, contagious disease, it is not spread in the same manner as a common cold or chicken pox. It is not spread by sneezing or coughing, as are airborne illnesses. HIV is not spread by sharing a bathroom, swimming in a pool, or by hugging or shaking hands. Studies of family members who lived with and cared for AIDS patients have not found definitive evidence that anyone has become infected through casual contact. Still, myths abound. To combat misinformation, the U.S. Surgeon General's office and public health education initiatives continue to stress that HIV is *not* spread by:

- Bites from mosquitoes or other insects.

- Bites from animals.

- Food handled, prepared, or served by HIV-infected people.

- Forks, spoons, knives, or drinking glasses used by HIV-infected people.

- Chairs previously occupied by people with HIV.

- Casual contact such as touching, hugging, or kissing a person who is HIV-positive (open-mouth kissing with a person who is HIV-positive is not recommended because of potential exposure to blood).

Donating Blood

Health officials agree that donating blood poses no danger of HIV infection for the donors. The needles used to draw blood from donors are new and are thrown away after one use. Contact with HIV from donating blood is therefore impossible.

SAFETY OF BLOOD AND TRANSPLANT PROCEDURES

According to the CDC, more than 400 American institutions either bank or commercially process one or more human tissues, organs, or fluids. Approximately one hundred eye banks, 125 bone banks, one hundred semen banks, ninety-nine bone marrow transplant centers, and seven human milk banks operate in the United States. Additionally, the number of hospitals that store bone and the number of physicians' offices that store semen is undetermined and likely large.

To safeguard the nation's transplant recipients, the CDC suggests that all donors of blood products, tissue, and organs be screened and tested. The recommendations include screening for behaviors—risk factors—associated with the acquisition of HIV infection, a physical examination for signs and symptoms related to HIV infection, and laboratory screening for antibodies to HIV. It is important to remember that the CDC does not regulate medical protocol; its main function is to offer health care guidelines and information to the nation and its health care providers.

The U.S. Blood Supply

Before HIV-antibody testing began in 1985, it is estimated that 70% of hemophiliacs (people with inherited bleeding disorders) who received blood products were given tainted blood-clotting factor (a concentrate of blood used to stem bleeding) and were therefore infected with HIV. Approximately ten thousand of these patients developed AIDS and, according to the National Hemophilia Foundation, most have died.

Widespread use of two blood-screening tests, both of which are also used on plasma and other blood products, has strengthened the safety of the U.S. blood and plasma supply. Since 1992 the Public Health Service, an arm of the U.S. Department of Health and Human Services, has required that all blood and plasma donations be screened for the rare HIV-2 antibody, as well as the more common HIV-1 antibody.

In 2001 the FDA approved the first nucleic acid test (NAT) system to screen plasma donors for HIV. Rather than relying on the identification of antigens or antibodies, the new test provides extremely sensitive detection of RNA from HIV-1. Even with the new test, however, there is still some risk due to the "window period" during which a person who has acquired the HIV-1 infection may still test negative. For HIV-1 antigen and antibody detection, the window period is sixteen and twenty-two days, respectively, following infection. NAT systems reduce the window period to twelve days. Put another way, anyone who is infected with HIV and who donates blood more than twelve days after exposure to the virus will register HIV-positive.

Of the twelve million units of blood donated annually in the United States, the CDC estimates that between thirty-two and forty-nine units are potentially infectious. While the U.S. blood supply is considered safe, blood banks across the country nonetheless encourage individuals concerned about tainted blood to bank their own blood for possible future use.

Foreign Blood Supplies

HIV infection from contaminated blood has been much more common in other countries. In July 1998 a French court ruled that a former prime minister and two former cabinet members would be tried on charges that they allowed HIV-contaminated blood to be used for transfusions during 1984 and 1985. Relatives of the patients argued that the French government had refused American technology that would have detected antibodies in the tainted blood in favor of a French procedure in development. Estimates vary, but as many as four thousand people acquired HIV as a result of this action. An estimated 1,250 hemophiliacs were infected and at least 400 of them, including many children, have since died of AIDS. The former French officials, Prime Minister Laurent Fabius, Social Affairs Minister Georgina Dufoix, and Health Minister Edmond Herve, faced charges of involuntary homicide and went to trial in 1999. Herve was

convicted without a penalty and Dufoix and Fabius were acquitted. The tragedy resulted in the overhaul of the blood supply and donation networks in France.

In 1995 the WHO reported that three thousand children in Romania—home to thousands of abandoned babies left in squalid institutions after the fall of Romanian dictator Nicolae Ceausescu—were infected by contaminated blood and syringes in the late 1980s. The WHO estimates that one thousand of those children have died. In 1998 Romania had more than half of the juvenile AIDS cases in Europe; more than 90% of the country's AIDS cases were among children. The Romanian Health Ministry faced litigation for causing the spread of HIV.

In 1995 the owner of a German drug laboratory was charged with nearly six thousand counts of murder or attempted murder for selling HIV-tainted blood products to German hospitals in 1987. Not all of the six thousand batches distributed had been tested for HIV. Testing has been mandatory in Germany since 1986.

The Canadian blood collection, testing, and distribution system was completely overhauled in the wake of the distribution of HIV-contaminated blood before 1986 (when HIV testing was not yet available) and after 1990 (when more sensitive tests that could detect HIV were available, but which were not immediately used by the Canadian blood collection service). In 2001 Canada's Supreme Court ruled that the negligence of the blood agency during the early years of the AIDS crisis entitled several thousand affected Canadians to a $1.2 billion federal-provincial government compensation offer. Legal wrangling in the intervening years has delayed the implementation of the court's ruling. As of June 2005, those affected by the tainted blood have yet to be financially compensated.

Organ and Tissue Transplants

In several instances HIV has been transmitted through organ (kidney, liver, heart, lung, and pancreas) and other tissue transplants. The risk of such transmission is low simply because there are far fewer transplant cases than blood transfusions.

In 1994 the FDA began regulating the sale of bone, skin, corneas, cartilage, tendons, and similar nonblood vessel-bearing tissues used for transplants. The FDA requires that all procurement agencies conduct behavioral screening and infectious-disease (HIV-1, HIV-2, hepatitis B virus, and hepatitis C virus) testing of donors.

TESTING PEOPLE FOR HIV

A person infected with HIV produces antibodies specific to the virus as part of the body's immune response to the invader. While the antibodies are not enough to successfully fight HIV, they are of diagnostic value, as they can indicate the presence of the virus.

Antibody-based HIV testing is done, rather than a direct test for the virus itself, because it is too difficult to isolate the virus from the blood. Testing serves to determine if there is a viral infection in donated blood, tissues, or organs. This protects the recipients of the donated material and can be used to identify HIV-infected donors.

An antibody-based test cannot detect all HIV-positive blood. It can typically take between four and twelve weeks following HIV infection for antibodies to appear, although in rare cases this period can be up to one year. This interval between acquisition of the virus and the appearance of antibodies is called the "window period." The introduction of tests that detect the viral nucleic acid rather than the HIV antibodies has markedly increased the detection sensitivity of blood screening. Still, even nucleic acid detection has a window period, albeit a shorter one, of about twelve days.

The fact that detection is not absolute from the moment of HIV infection means that the possibility exists that some HIV-infected donors may not be diagnosed and their blood may enter the nation's blood supply. However, the number of predicted contaminated blood samples is extremely small. To try to further reduce the chances of contaminated blood entering the blood supply, blood banks routinely question potential donors about high-risk behaviors. Any donor whose behavior might indicate an increased risk of HIV infection (such as intravenous drug use or male-to-male sex) is automatically excluded from donating blood.

Diagnostic Tools for HIV Antibodies

Two tests commonly used to detect HIV antibodies are believed to be about 99% reliable. These tests are the enzyme-linked immunosorbent assay (ELISA) and the Western blot.

ELISA, introduced in 1985, is a test designed for screening rather than diagnosing. The assay uses purified HIV antigens to probe for the presence of complimentary antibodies in a sample such as blood. If anti-HIV antibodies are present in the sample, they attach themselves to the viral proteins that have been immobilized on a plastic surface. A second antibody that has been raised against the anti-HIV antibody (antibodies are proteins too, and so can themselves function as antigens, stimulating the formation of antibodies) is bound to the anti-HIV antibodies. The second antibody also contains a chemical that can be made to change color. The color change reveals the presence of the anti-HIV antibody. If no color change appears, no anti-HIV antibody is present in the blood sample. This test is reliable, simple to conduct, and inexpensive.

The Western blot, introduced in 1987, is a confirmatory test. This means the test is commonly used to verify the results of the less-specific assays. The Western blot

technique separates the various HIV proteins from one another, based on their speed of movement through a gel under the influence of electricity. The separated proteins are transferred from the gel to a membrane made of a material such as nitrocellulose. When the nitrocellulose is exposed to a blood sample, antibodies that recognize one of the proteins on the nitrocellulose will bind to the particular protein. As with ELISA, a color reaction can be induced to indicate the site of the bound antibodies. The Western blot provides a positive, negative, or intermediate result. The presence of three or more of the color bands confirms an HIV infection. If fewer—one or two—bands appear, the test is considered intermediate and retesting is performed six months later. If no color bands appear, the test is considered negative with no HIV present, though many people who test negative also repeat the test six months later.

Urine Tests

In June 1998 the FDA approved a new, urine-based diagnostic kit for HIV marketed by Calypte Biomedical Corporation that does not require confirmation by blood test. Urine tests are easier to use and cost less than blood tests for health care providers. According to the National Institutes of Health, there is no evidence that HIV is spread through urine. Therefore, the chances of accidental infection through needle sticks or handling of samples are lessened. The urine test and its urine-based confirmation test, like most blood tests, recognize the existence of antibodies, not the actual virus.

The test is marketed to life insurance companies, clinical laboratories, public health agencies, the military, immigration authorities, and the criminal justice system. In June 2000 Calypte announced its partnership with the Chinese National Center for AIDS Prevention and Control (NCAIDS) to distribute the first HIV-1 antibody urine test in the People's Republic of China. NCAIDS estimates that the total number of HIV infections in China could rise to as high as ten million before 2010 if proper countermeasures are not taken.

A clinical trial of Calypte's diagnostic kit for HIV was conducted by the Chinese CDC, involving approximately fifteen hundred people, some known to be HIV-positive and some uninfected. Results released in early September 2005 indicated the kits were successful, and Calypte planned on submitting the kits for approval in China, which plans to use the product as the exclusive noninvasive method of testing for HIV.

Home Testing

In 1997 a recently approved home HIV test was analyzed in a multisite test study involving 1,255 people. Test participants registered anonymously by telephone with a testing laboratory. The subjects simply stuck a finger to draw blood and mailed the dried blood sample on filter paper to the laboratory. There, a phlebotomist (a health worker who draws blood by syringe or needle) matched the results with blood that had been drawn earlier from the patient's vein in the traditional manner. Results of the test were obtained by calling a toll-free telephone number. Negative results were given by recorded message. For positive results, a trained counselor offered callers follow-up information and counseling. Of the 1,255 people who participated, 1,104 participants called in to check their test results. For those participants the home test matched the phlebotomy results exactly.

Although there is no new technology involved in home testing, it offers the advantages of privacy and ease of use. Critics of home testing point out that it is expensive; a kit costs $40 to $60 and may be prohibitively expensive for poorer populations—for whom such a test is most needed. Critics also question the impersonal practice of relaying HIV-positive results and follow-up counseling by telephone.

As of 2005 the FDA had approved only the Home Access Express HIV Test System, produced by the Home Access Health Corporation. The FDA warned that non-approved home HIV tests could produce inaccurate results. When Home Access testing kits were made available over the counter, rather than by physician prescription, in 1998, sales at two retail drugstore chains that were surveyed increased 360 to 570%.

Quick-Response Tests

During the mid- to late 1990s, the CDC recommended the development of a new HIV test that would give results instantly. The CDC hoped that this would encourage people to learn the results of their tests. Currently, nearly seven hundred thousand people each year do not follow up to learn their test results. The CDC stresses the importance of obtaining results quickly. They contend that people are not only more likely to take a test that gives results instantly, but will also benefit from the opportunity to learn they are infected before their immune systems have been seriously damaged. Furthermore, rapid results may lead to earlier, more effective treatment and might reduce transmission of the virus.

The FDA has approved a number of rapid tests designed for use in clinics in the United States. The first test to be approved is manufactured by Murex Diagnostics Inc. of Norcross, Georgia. This test detects the presence of HIV antibody in about ten minutes. The test is as accurate as the standard Western blot test. But because the Western blot test also looks for protein bands, this test remains the absolute antibody-based indicator of HIV.

In late 2002 the FDA announced approval of another blood-based antibody test (OraQuick Rapid HIV-1 by OraSure Technologies Inc., Bethlehem, Pennsylvania) for use. As of 2005 the test, which produces results within about ten minutes, is not licensed for home use and can only be performed in a clinical setting. But the fact that the test does not require any specialized equipment or refrigeration offers the possibility of home use in the future.

Another similar rapid test kit, developed and manufactured by MedMira Inc. of Halifax, Canada, was granted FDA approval in April 2003 for sale in the United States. The kit is also approved in China, where HIV infection rates dramatically increased in the early 2000s.

Rapid HIV tests are used more frequently in other countries, such as China. In developing countries, for example, quick-response tests are used to screen blood before transfusions, to screen pregnant women so medical interventions can be given to prevent mother-to-child transmission of the virus, and in rural clinics.

Test Tracks HIV/AIDS Progression

In June 1996 the FDA approved a test to help determine how fast an HIV infection progressed to full-blown AIDS. Developed by Roche Diagnostic Systems Inc., the Amplicor HIV-1 monitor test is not intended to screen for HIV or to confirm an HIV diagnosis. Instead, the test detects the amount of HIV in the blood (the viral load) by measuring HIV genetic material. An increased viral load indicates the advancement of the infection toward AIDS and an increasing predisposition to the development of OIs. The test is based on a technique developed in 1984 called the polymerase chain reaction (PCR). PCR uses a heat-resistant bacterial enzyme to amplify the copies of target stretches of genetic material to detectable amounts. The process can be completed in less than one hour. This test was the first PCR-based test to be approved.

In 1997 FDA approval was granted to expand the use of the test as an aid in managing HIV in patients undergoing antiretroviral therapy. In 1999 a more sensitive version of the test became available. As of 2005 the test was used in eight out of ten clinical labs worldwide, according to the manufacturer.

CHAPTER 3

PATTERNS AND TRENDS IN HIV/AIDS SURVEILLANCE

DETERMINING THE NUMBER OF PEOPLE INFECTED WITH HIV

The Centers for Disease Control and Prevention (CDC), headquartered in Atlanta, Georgia, keeps track of the number of people in the United States who are infected with HIV, the virus that is generally acknowledged to be the cause of AIDS.

These CDC figures—which have always been acknowledged as estimates—have been criticized as being either too high or too low. Nonetheless, the historical continuity of the agency's data allows trend analyses to be done. Therefore, when viewed over a number of years, the figures provide a reasonable indication of the progress of the disease in the United States.

Estimates of HIV infection are important, as they directly influence public health, medical resource allocation, and political and economic decisions. Definitive figures are difficult to obtain because laws prevent testing for HIV without consent and permission. Furthermore, many people are understandably reluctant to participate in household surveys because of confidentiality concerns and fear of losing or failing to get insurance coverage.

Health officials contend that knowing the prevalence of HIV infections (prevalence is a measure of all cases of illness existing at a given point in time) is not as crucial as knowing whether the number of HIV infections is rising or falling. The rate at which people develop HIV/AIDS during a specified period of time is known as the incidence rate. Since there are no national studies to collect this data (not all states require reporting of new HIV cases), estimates are based on reports from states that mandate confidential reporting of HIV cases, along with other small studies and surveys. Officials with the CDC explain that a major problem has been the lack of knowledge about how many people have become infected prior to the beginning of the agency's regular collection of data. This would help to determine how the current incidence of HIV compares to previous years. Comparison of incidence rates is important because they are a direct measure of the rate at which individuals become ill and provide data to help estimate the risk or probability of illness.

The CDC data through December 2003 from the thirty-three states with confidential HIV reporting and adjusted estimates from reported cases in other states found that 174,639 people were living with HIV that have not yet progressed to AIDS. (See Table 3.1.) This is an increase from 127,058 reported through December 2000 and 161,976 as of December 2001. Of the 2003 total, 1,687 were children younger than thirteen years old (a drop from 2,905 in 2001) and 172,952 were adults and adolescents (an increase from 158,806 in 2001).

The CDC also compiles figures on the numbers of people living with AIDS. Through December 2003, 403,928 adults and adolescents were estimated to be living with AIDS, an increase from the reported 331,471 adults and adolescents through 2001. The number of children younger than thirteen living with AIDS through 2003 (1,942) was a drop from the 2,410 children through 2001. The December 2003 data also indicate that among U.S. territories, a total of 10,131 people were living with AIDS, an increase from the 10,096 reported through 2001. This total includes fifty-one children younger than thirteen (a decrease from eighty-two through 2001) and 10,080 adults and adolescents (9,749 through 2001).

AIDS CASE NUMBERS

The first cases of what came to be recognized as AIDS were reported in the United States in June 1981. Five young, homosexual males in Los Angeles were diagnosed with *Pneumocystis carinii* pneumonia and other opportunistic infections. By August 1989 approximately one hundred thousand cases of AIDS had been reported to the CDC. By December 1997 that

TABLE 3.1

Estimated numbers of persons living with HIV infection or AIDS, by state or area of residence and age category, December 2003

Area of residence	Living with HIV infection (not AIDS)[a]			Living with AIDS		
	Adults or adolescents	Children <13 years old	Total	Adults or adolescents	Children <13 years old	Total
Alabama	5,863	33	5,896	3,924	15	3,940
Alaska	262	0	261	269	2	271
Arizona	5,452	41	5,493	4,122	5	4,127
Arkansas	2,281	13	2,294	2,057	10	2,067
California	—	—	—	55,612	138	55,750
Colorado	6,118	14	6,132	3,672	3	3,675
Connecticut	—	—	—	6,959	30	6,989
Delaware	—	—	—	1,601	12	1,613
District of Columbia	—	—	—	8,785	63	8,848
Florida[b]	32,196	253	32,449	42,861	361	43,223
Georgia	—	—	—	13,963	60	14,023
Hawaii	—	—	—	1,314	4	1,318
Idaho	389	1	390	274	0	274
Illinois	—	—	—	14,241	80	14,321
Indiana	3,874	29	3,902	3,668	18	3,686
Iowa	469	4	473	725	3	728
Kansas	1,133	9	1,143	1,120	3	1,123
Kentucky	—	—	—	2,349	10	2,359
Louisiana	7,675	98	7,773	7,549	43	7,592
Maine	—	—	—	515	3	518
Maryland	—	—	—	12,830	81	12,911
Massachusetts	—	—	—	8,362	35	8,397
Michigan	5,799	72	5,871	5,562	22	5,584
Minnesota	3,136	24	3,160	1,890	10	1,900
Mississippi	4,341	34	4,375	2,856	19	2,875
Missouri	4,881	39	4,920	5,046	14	5,060
Montana	—	—	—	175	0	175
Nebraska	594	6	600	594	4	598
Nevada	3,377	15	3,392	2,648	6	2,654
New Hampshire	—	—	—	526	3	530
New Jersey	15,192	294	15,487	16,969	119	17,089
New Mexico	816	0	816	1,178	4	1,182
New York	—	—	—	66,311	349	66,660
North Carolina	11,118	86	11,204	6,519	25	6,545
North Dakota	72	1	73	56	1	57
Ohio	7,585	66	7,651	6,548	35	6,583
Oklahoma	2,615	18	2,633	2,081	4	2,085
Oregon	—	—	—	2,579	6	2,586
Pennsylvania	—	—	—	15,054	123	15,178
Rhode Island	—	—	—	1,093	10	1,103
South Carolina	6,906	64	6,970	6,349	29	6,379
South Dakota	197	2	199	104	1	105
Tennessee	6,612	66	6,678	5,806	11	5,817
Texas	20,820	305	21,125	29,958	85	30,043
Utah	687	9	696	1,098	0	1,098
Vermont	—	—	—	247	3	250
Virginia	9,182	60	9,242	7,682	53	7,735
Washington	—	—	—	5,102	6	5,108
West Virginia	686	5	690	640	5	645
Wisconsin	2,297	19	2,316	1,837	11	1,848
Wyoming	89	1	90	95	1	96
Subtotal	172,714	1,683	174,396	393,375	1,942	395,317

number had risen to 641,086; of these, 390,692 people had died. As of December 2001 the total of all reported cases was 788,672; 467,910 of these people had died. Cumulatively through 2003 there were 872,629 reported cases of AIDS in the United States; 524,060 people had died of the disease. (See Table 3.2 and Table 3.3.)

During the mid-1990s the number of AIDS cases rose dramatically. This surge was not an actual numerical increase, but was due to the expanded 1993 AIDS surveillance definition, which added diseases and conditions that had not been part of the prior definition of AIDS. By the late 1990s the number of AIDS cases leveled off and began to decline, probably as a result of the increasing use of effective antiretroviral drugs that delay the progression of AIDS. The number of new cases reported between December 2001 and December 2003 (83,957, representing an annual average of 41,979) was higher than the 31,682 new cases reported between December 2000 and

TABLE 3.1

Estimated numbers of persons living with HIV infection or AIDS, by state or area of residence and age category, December 2003 [CONTINUED]

	Living with HIV infection (not AIDS)[a]			Living with AIDS		
Area of residence	Adults or adolescents	Children <13 years old	Total	Adults or adolescents	Children <13 years old	Total
U.S. dependencies, possessions, and associated nations						
Guam	—	—	—	36	0	35
Pacific Islands, U.S.	—	—	—	4	0	4
Puerto Rico	—	—	—	9,748	49	9,798
Virgin Islands, U.S.	238	4	243	292	2	294
Total[c]	**172,952**	**1,687**	**174,639**	**403,928**	**1,998**	**405,926**

Note: These numbers do not represent reported case counts. Rather, these numbers are point estimates, which result from adjustments of reported case counts. The reported case counts are adjusted for reporting delays. The estimates do not include adjustment for incomplete reporting. Age category is based on age as of end of 2003.
Since 1999, the following 33 areas have had laws or regulations requiring confidential name-based HIV infection reporting: Alabama, Alaska, Arizona, Arkansas, Colorado, Florida, Idaho, Indiana, Iowa, Kansas, Louisiana, Michigan, Minnesota, Mississippi, Missouri, Nebraska, Nevada, New Jersey, New Mexico, North Carolina, North Dakota, Ohio, Oklahoma, South Carolina, South Dakota, Tennessee, Texas, Utah, Virginia, West Virginia, Wisconsin, Wyoming, and the U.S. Virgin Islands. Since July 1997, Florida has had confidential name-based HIV infection reporting only for new diagnoses.
[a]Includes only persons living with HIV infection that has not progressed to AIDS.
[b]Florida (since July 1997) has had confidential name-based HIV infection reporting only for new diagnoses.
[c]Total number of persons living with HIV infection (not AIDS) includes persons reported from areas with confidential name-based HIV infection reporting who were residents of other states or whose area of residence is unknown. Total number of persons living with AIDS includes persons whose area of residence is unknown. Because column totals were calculated independently of the values for the subpopulations, the values in each column may not sum to the column total.

SOURCE: "Table 12. Estimated Numbers of Persons Living with HIV Infection (Not AIDS) or with AIDS at the End of 2003, by State or Area of Residence and Age Category," in *HIV/AIDS Surveillance Report: Cases of HIV Infection and AIDS in the United States, 2003*, vol. 15, Centers for Disease Control and Prevention, 2004, http://www.cdc.gov/hiv/stats/2003SurveillanceReport.pdf (accessed July 18, 2005)

December 2001, but lower than the 42,156 new cases reported from December 1999 through December 2000, which in turn was lower than the 47,083 cases reported in the period from December 1998 through December 1999.

THE NATURE OF THE EPIDEMIC

The changes in the distribution of HIV illustrate the increasing diversity of those affected by the epidemic in the more than twenty years since AIDS was first diagnosed. In 1981 all of the 189 AIDS cases reported in the United States were males. Three-fourths of these were men who have sex with men (in the 2003 CDC surveys, this category has been changed to male-to-male sexual contact, or MTM) living in New York and California. In 1990, of the more than 43,000 AIDS cases reported by all states, approximately 30% were from New York and California, 11% were women, and about 2% were children. In 1999 the proportions of reported cases among women, African-Americans, Hispanics, and people exposed through heterosexual contact all increased. On the other hand, the percentage of reported cases among whites and MTM declined somewhat.

Regional Differences

AIDS cases have been reported in all fifty states, the District of Columbia, and four U.S. territories. But the distribution of cases is far from even. In 2003 the annual adult and adolescent AIDS incidence rates per one hundred thousand population in the United States and U.S. possession and territories (see Figure 3.1) varied from 10.5 in North Dakota to 1,833.2 in the District of Columbia (the same pattern was evident from 1999 to 2000). Most recently reported cases show a concentration on the East Coast (particularly Connecticut, Maryland, New Jersey, and Delaware, with respective rates of 243.9, 284.4, 239.3, and 235.6, and Florida, with a rate of 301.9). Also prominent were Puerto Rico (rate of 316.6) and the U.S. Virgin Islands (rate of 345.4). Figure 3.2 shows the corresponding HIV and AIDS rates for children younger than thirteen in 2003.

RATES IN MAJOR METROPOLITAN AREAS. The majority of AIDS cases are concentrated in larger metropolitan regions (the city and surrounding suburbs). Metropolitan areas with populations of five hundred thousand or more accounted for 81% of all reported cases between 2000 and 2001 and 84% of the cumulative totals since 1981 (cumulative totals include both those who have died and those still living). In 2002 and 2003 the metropolitan AIDS incidence rates per one hundred thousand people were highest on the coasts, such as in New York City (60.1 and 59.2, respectively), Miami (49.2 and 45.8), Baltimore (48.4 and 39.3), Jersey City, New Jersey (32.6 and 28.3), Fort Lauderdale, Florida (44.0 and 39.9), West Palm Beach, Florida (48.1 and 36.7), Baton Rouge, Louisiana (49.4 and 33.7), Newark, New Jersey (27.6 and 25.8), Columbia, South Carolina (37.0 and 33.5), and San Francisco (31.9 and 45.2). On the other hand, Midwest metropolitan areas displayed the lowest rates: Akron, Ohio (4.1 and 3.4), Grand Rapids, Michigan (4.7 and 4.4), and Youngstown, Ohio (4.1 and 4.3).

TABLE 3.2

Estimated numbers of deaths of persons with AIDS, by year of death and selected characteristics, 1999–2003

	Year of death					Cumulative through 2003[a]
	1999	**2000**	**2001**	**2002**	**2003**	
Age at death (years)						
<13	97	51	48	35	29	5,103
13–14	18	8	4	11	8	252
15–24	232	216	270	199	229	9,789
25–34	3,258	2,823	2,512	2,143	1,928	142,761
35–44	7,706	7,138	7,525	6,896	6,970	216,093
45–54	4,994	5,203	5,548	5,737	5,964	104,064
55–64	1,556	1,631	1,873	1,840	2,146	33,717
≥65	630	670	743	696	741	12,282
Race/ethnicity						
White, not Hispanic	5,834	5,559	5,524	5,128	4,767	230,289
Black, not Hispanic	9,106	8,832	9,345	8,923	9,048	195,891
Hispanic	3,341	3,162	3,435	3,274	3,915	92,370
Asian/Pacific Islander	113	103	108	94	85	3,340
American Indian/Alaska Native	79	67	83	79	78	1,529
Transmission category						
Male adult or adolescent						
Male-to-male sexual contact	6,703	6,316	6,479	6,012	6,015	257,898
Injection drug use	4,425	4,182	4,298	4,126	4,166	107,797
Male-to-male sexual contact and injection drug use	1,335	1,334	1,396	1,285	1,233	38,083
Heterosexual contact	1,403	1,417	1,585	1,526	1,644	23,080
Other[b]	194	204	174	166	140	9,846
Subtotal	14,061	13,454	13,932	13,116	13,198	436,704
Female adult or adolescent						
Injection drug use	2,051	1,925	1,985	1,956	2,056	39,848
Heterosexual contact	2,157	2,192	2,444	2,335	2,584	37,901
Other[b]	97	92	92	89	95	4,115
Subtotal	4,305	4,209	4,521	4,379	4,736	81,864
Child (<13 yrs at diagnosis)						
Perinatal	117	72	67	58	78	4,961
Other[c]	8	5	4	4	5	531
Subtotal	124	78	71	62	83	5,492
Region of residence						
Northeast	5,698	5,294	5,344	5,015	6,140	168,213
Midwest	1,712	1,685	1,839	1,550	1,343	50,258
South	7,406	7,352	7,624	7,526	7,068	178,447
West	2,952	2,681	2,817	2,520	2,588	107,767
U.S. dependencies, possessions, and associated nations	723	729	900	947	877	19,375
Total[d]	**18,491**	**17,741**	**18,524**	**17,557**	**18,017**	**524,060**

Note: These numbers do not represent reported case counts. Rather, these numbers are point estimates, which result from adjustments of reported case counts. The reported case counts are adjusted for reporting delays and for redistribution of cases in persons initially reported without an identified risk factor. The estimates do not include adjustment for incomplete reporting.

[a]Includes persons who died with AIDS, from the beginning of the epidemic through 2003.
[b]Includes hemophilia, blood transfusion, perinatal, and risk factor not reported or not identified.
[c]Includes hemophilia, blood transfusion, and risk factor not reported or not identified.
[d]Includes persons of unknown race or multiple races and persons of unknown sex. Cumulative total includes 640 persons of unknown race or multiple races. Because column totals were calculated independently of the values for the subpopulations, the values in each column may not sum to the column total.

SOURCE: "Table 7. Estimated Numbers of Deaths of Persons with AIDS, by Year of Death and Selected Characteristics, 1999–2003—United States," in *HIV/AIDS Surveillance Report: Cases of HIV Infection and AIDS in the United States, 2003*, vol. 15, Centers for Disease Control and Prevention, 2004, http://www.cdc.gov/hiv/stats/2003SurveillanceReport.pdf (accessed July 18, 2005)

Ann Arbor, Michigan, had the lowest overall metropolitan rate (3.0 and 3.3), followed by Salt Lake City, Utah (3.8 and 4.3), and Scranton, Pennsylvania (3.9 and 5.4). (See Table 3.4.)

There are several reasons for the higher rates in urban areas. First, metropolitan areas are more cosmopolitan and, by definition, more tolerant of alternative lifestyles such as those of MTM, a group with high-risk sexual behaviors. Second, large metropolitan areas also have greater numbers of intravenous drug users (IDUs), another major risk factor for HIV infection. Third, while HIV infection and transmission are not restricted to more populated areas, those who need and seek treatment may

TABLE 3.3

Reported AIDS cases and annual rates, by area of residence and age category, cumulative through 2003

Area of residence	2002		2003		Cumulative through 2003[a]		
	No.	Rate	No.	Rate	Adults or adolescents	Children (<13 years)	Total
Alabama	433	9.7	472	10.5	7,531	76	7,607
Alaska	35	5.5	23	3.5	559	6	565
Arizona	633	11.6	614	11.0	9,166	42	9,208
Arkansas	239	8.8	188	6.9	3,543	38	3,581
California	4,228	12.1	5,903	16.6	132,650	642	133,292
Colorado	326	7.2	366	8.0	8,042	31	8,073
Connecticut	611	17.7	736	21.1	13,284	180	13,464
Delaware	193	23.9	213	26.1	3,206	25	3,231
District of Columbia	926	162.7	961	170.6	15,660	181	15,841
Florida	4,979	29.8	4,666	27.4	93,235	1,490	94,725
Georgia	1,471	17.2	1,907	22.0	27,697	218	27,915
Hawaii	131	10.6	110	8.7	2,816	17	2,833
Idaho	31	2.3	26	1.9	569	3	572
Illinois	2,111	16.8	1,730	13.7	29,857	282	30,139
Indiana	491	8.0	507	8.2	7,450	54	7,504
Iowa	90	3.1	77	2.6	1,554	13	1,567
Kansas	71	2.6	116	4.3	2,647	12	2,659
Kentucky	304	7.4	219	5.3	4,162	30	4,192
Louisiana	1,163	26.0	1,041	23.2	15,519	134	15,653
Maine	28	2.2	52	4.0	1,075	9	1,084
Maryland	1,848	33.9	1,570	28.5	26,606	312	26,918
Massachusetts	808	12.6	757	11.8	18,311	214	18,525
Michigan	795	7.9	680	6.7	13,215	111	13,326
Minnesota	162	3.2	177	3.5	4,225	27	4,252
Mississippi	436	15.2	508	17.6	5,742	57	5,799
Missouri	388	6.8	403	7.1	10,346	60	10,406
Montana	17	1.9	7	0.8	363	3	366
Nebraska	71	4.1	59	3.4	1,286	10	1,296
Nevada	313	14.4	277	12.4	5,209	28	5,237
New Hampshire	39	3.1	37	2.9	985	10	995
New Jersey	1,456	17.0	1,516	17.5	45,936	767	46,703
New Mexico	86	4.6	109	5.8	2,381	8	2,389
New York	6,741	35.2	6,684	34.8	160,109	2,337	162,446
North Carolina	1,045	12.6	1,083	12.9	13,335	121	13,456
North Dakota	3	0.5	3	0.5	114	1	115
Ohio	773	6.8	775	6.8	13,373	129	13,502
Oklahoma	205	5.9	213	6.1	4,414	27	4,441
Oregon	300	8.5	242	6.8	5,580	19	5,599
Pennsylvania	1,789	14.5	1,895	15.3	29,639	349	29,988
Rhode Island	107	10.0	102	9.5	2,337	26	2,363
South Carolina	822	20.0	774	18.7	11,724	94	11,818
South Dakota	11	1.4	13	1.7	214	4	218
Tennessee	772	13.3	837	14.3	10,686	54	10,740
Texas	3,076	14.2	3,379	15.3	62,592	391	62,983
Utah	68	2.9	73	3.1	2,156	20	2,176
Vermont	12	1.9	16	2.6	451	6	457
Virginia	948	13.0	777	10.5	15,544	179	15,723
Washington	471	7.8	525	8.6	10,953	34	10,987
West Virginia	82	4.5	94	5.2	1,341	11	1,352
Wisconsin	187	3.4	184	3.4	4,103	33	4,136
Wyoming	11	2.2	8	1.6	210	2	212
Subtotal	42,336	14.7	43,704	15.0	863,702	8,927	872,629
U.S. dependencies, possessions, and associated nations							
Guam	2	1.2	6	3.7	64	1	65
Pacific Islands, U.S.	0	0.0	1	0.7	2	0	2
Puerto Rico	1,135	29.4	1,065	27.5	27,903	398	28,301
Virgin Islands	54	49.6	34	31.2	585	18	603
Total[b]	**43,578**	**14.9**	**44,963**	**15.2**	**892,875**	**9,348**	**902,223**

[a]Includes persons with a diagnosis of AIDS, reported from the beginning of the epidemic through 2003.
[b]Includes persons whose state or area of residence is unknown. Cumulative total includes 620 persons whose state or area of residence is unknown.

SOURCE: "Table 14. Reported AIDS Cases and Annual Rates (per 100,000 Population), by Area of Residence and Age Category, Cumulative through 2003—United States," in *HIV/AIDS Surveillance Report: Cases of HIV Infection and AIDS in the United States, 2003*, vol. 15, Centers for Disease Control and Prevention, 2004, http://www.cdc.gov/hiv/stats/2003SurveillanceReport.pdf (accessed July 18, 2005)

FIGURE 3.1

Estimated rates for adults and adolescents living with HIV infection or AIDS, 2003

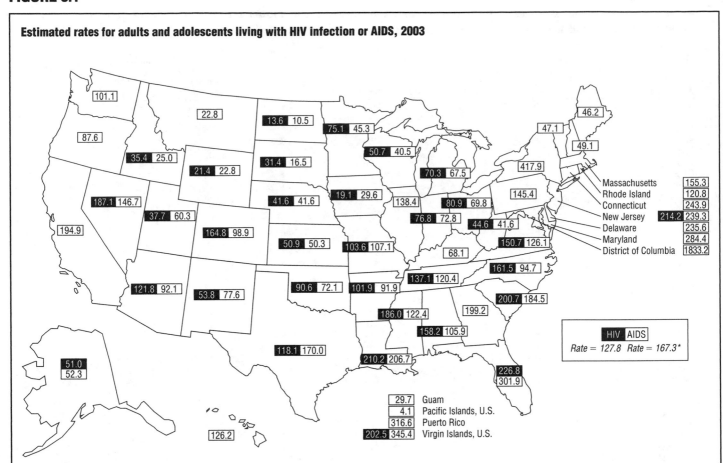

Massachusetts `155.3`
Rhode Island `120.8`
Connecticut `243.9`
New Jersey `214.2` `239.3`
Delaware `235.6`
Maryland `284.4`
District of Columbia `1833.2`

HIV AIDS
Rate = 127.8 Rate = 167.3*

`29.7` Guam
`4.1` Pacific Islands, U.S.
`316.6` Puerto Rico
`202.5` `345.4` Virgin Islands, U.S.

Note. Rates adjusted for reporting delays. Rates of HIV infection include only persons living with HIV infection that has not progressed to AIDS.
Since 1999, the following 33 areas with laws or regulations requiring confidential name-based HIV infection reporting: Alabama, Alaska, Arizona, Arkansas, Colorado, Florida, Idaho, Indiana, Iowa, Kansas, Louisiana, Michigan, Minnesota, Mississippi, Missouri, Nebraska, Nevada, New Jersey, New Mexico, North Carolina, North Dakota, Ohio, Oklahoma, South Carolina, South Dakota, Tennessee, Texas, Utah, Virginia, West Virginia, Wisconsin, Wyoming, and the U.S. Virgin Islands.
*Includes persons whose area of residence is unknown.

SOURCE: "Map 1. Estimated Rates for Adults and Adolescents Living with HIV Infection (Not AIDS) or with AIDS (per 100,000 Population), 2003—United States," in *HIV/AIDS Surveillance Report: Cases of HIV Infection and AIDS in the United States, 2003*, vol. 15, Centers for Disease Control and Prevention, 2004, http://www.cdc.gov/hiv/stats/2003SurveillanceReport.pdf (accessed July 18, 2005)

migrate to these areas for access to medical care and social services. In many smaller communities medical care may be unavailable and financial and/or social barriers may limit access to health care services.

Rates among MTM: A Decline?

Table 3.5 displays CDC data on reported AIDS cases by age category, transmission category, and sex. The CDC reported 44,811 new adult and adolescent AIDS cases from January through December 2003, an increase from the 42,983 and 41,960 cases during the same periods in 2001 and 2000, respectively. Of the 2003 total, 33,250 were adult and adolescent males (compared with 31,901 in 2001 and 31,501 in 2000). Of these males, the portion attributable to transmission among MTM who did not also inject drugs was 15,859 cases (48% of total) in 2003, representing an increase from the 13,265 cases (42%) in 2001 and 13,562 cases (43%) in 2000. Since an

additional 4,866 (15%) of MTM in 2003, 1,502 (5%) in 2001, and 1,548 MTM (5%) in 2000 also used intravenous drugs, it is unclear whether AIDS was acquired from sexual behavior or intravenous drug use. Examination of data from 1981 (when record keeping began) until December 2003 reveals that men in the MTM exposure category who did not use intravenous drugs accounted for 55% of all men who had acquired AIDS and 45% of all reported AIDS cases. This latter percentage is slightly less than the cumulative 46% in both 2001 and 2000.

Rates among Women

In 2003 reported AIDS cases among women that were attributable to intravenous drug use (2,262) comprised 20% of the total number of cases (11,561), as compared with 2,212 cases in 2001 (20% of 11,082 cases). In 2000, 2,609 cases (25% of the total of

FIGURE 3.2

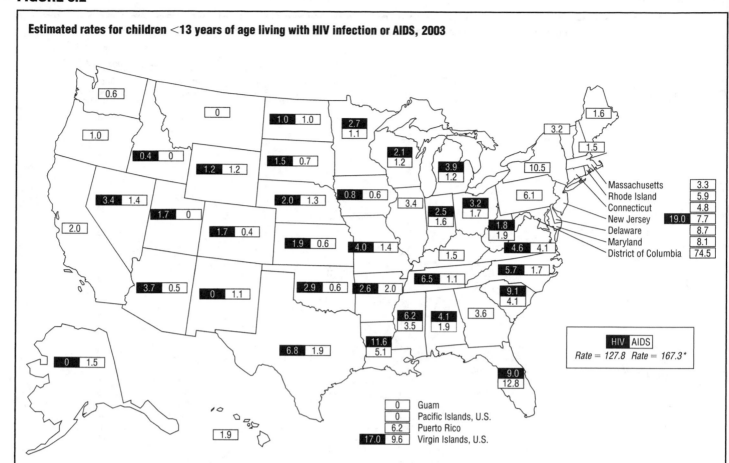

Estimated rates for children <13 years of age living with HIV infection or AIDS, 2003

	HIV	AIDS
Massachusetts		3.3
Rhode Island		5.9
Connecticut		4.8
New Jersey	19.0	7.7
Delaware		8.7
Maryland		8.1
District of Columbia		74.5

Rate = 127.8 | Rate = 167.3*

0	Guam	
0	Pacific Islands, U.S.	
6.2	Puerto Rico	
17.0 9.6	Virgin Islands, U.S.	

Note. Rates adjusted for reporting delays. Rates of HIV infection include only persons living with HIV infection that has not progressed to AIDS.
Since 1999, the following 33 areas with laws or regulations requiring confidential name-based HIV infection reporting: Alabama, Alaska, Arizona, Arkansas, Colorado, Florida, Idaho, Indiana, Iowa, Kansas, Louisiana, Michigan, Minnesota, Mississippi, Missouri, Nebraska, Nevada, New Jersey, New Mexico, North Carolina, North Dakota, Ohio, Oklahoma, South Carolina, South Dakota, Tennessee, Texas, Utah, Virginia, West Virginia, Wisconsin, Wyoming, and the U.S. Virgin Islands.
*Includes persons whose area of residence is unknown.

SOURCE: "Map 2. Estimated Rates for Children <13 Years of Age Living with HIV Infection (Not AIDS) or with AIDS (per 100,000 Population), 2003—United States," in *HIV/AIDS Surveillance Report: Cases of HIV Infection and AIDS in the United States, 2003*, vol. 15, Centers for Disease Control and Prevention, 2004, http://www.cdc.gov/hiv/stats/2003SurveillanceReport.pdf (accessed July 18, 2005)

10,459 cases) represented intravenous drug use. With respect to intravenous drug use, previous percentages were 23% in 1998 and 1999, and 19% in 1995. The actual number of cases remained fairly constant from 1994 to 1997—13,887 in 1994, 13,764 in 1995, 13,767 in 1996, and 13,105 in 1997—then dropping to 10,998 in 1998–99 and 10,459 in 2000 before increasing to 11,082 in 2001 and 11,561 in 2003. (See Table 3.5.)

When considering the role of heterosexual contact in the acquisition of AIDS, the proportion was far higher for women in 2003 (5,234 cases, representing 45% of the total of 11,561) than for men (3,371, representing 10% of the total of 40,947). Women with a history of heterosexual contact as their only risk factor made up 37% of all female cases in 2001. In contrast, 9% of men acquired HIV through heterosexual contact in 2001.

Decline in AIDS Due to Blood Transfusions

As a result of screening procedures for blood and blood products that began in 1985, the number of AIDS cases among adult and adolescent transfusion recipients decreased between 1995 (664 cases) and 1997 (409 cases). A pronounced decrease between 1998 and 1999 (266 cases) has been followed by 282 cases in 2000, 218 cases in 2001, and 219 in 2003. (See Table 3.5.)

The number of AIDS cases among adults and adolescents with hemophilia has also decreased. In 1996, 330 cases were reported. In 1997, 201 cases were reported. The number of new cases among hemophiliacs declined to 171 in 1999, 96 in 2000, 106 in 2001, and 85 in 2003. (See Table 3.5.)

Current Age and Gender Distribution

Of the 902,223 cumulative total reported cases of AIDS in 2003, 892,875 (99%) were among adults and

TABLE 3.4

Reported AIDS cases and annual rates, by metropolitan area of residence and age category, cumulative through 2003

Area of residence	2002		2003		Cumulative through 2003		
	No.	Rate	No.	Rate	Adults or adolescents	Children (<13 years)	Total
Akron, OH	29	4.1	24	3.4	659	1	660
Albany-Schenectady-Troy, NY	108	12.2	101	11.3	2,023	24	2,047
Albuquerque, NM	42	5.7	47	6.3	1,254	2	1,256
Allentown-Bethlehem-Easton, PA	54	8.3	82	12.4	1,043	13	1,056
Ann Arbor, MI	18	3.0	20	3.3	450	9	459
Atlanta, GA	1,015	23.2	1,212	27.1	19,248	121	19,369
Austin-San Marcos, TX	215	16.0	153	11.1	4,390	27	4,417
Bakersfield, CA	128	18.5	103	14.4	1,329	8	1,337
Baltimore, MD	1,257	48.4	1,028	39.3	17,833	214	18,047
Baton Rouge, LA	303	49.4	209	33.7	2,620	20	2,640
Bergen-Passaic, NJ	142	10.2	199	14.3	5,938	85	6,023
Birmingham, AL	115	12.3	127	13.5	2,237	23	2,260
Boston-Brocktn-Nashua, MA-NH Necma	721	11.7	664	10.8	16,100	190	16,290
Buffalo-Niagra Falls, NY	92	7.9	104	9.0	2,156	19	2,175
Charleston, SC	138	24.5	92	16.1	1,834	17	1,851
Charlotte-Gast.-Rock Hill, NC-SC	219	13.9	262	16.2	2,748	23	2,771
Chicago, IL	1,849	21.9	1,527	18.0	25,806	251	26,057
Cincinnati, OH-KY-IN	240	14.4	71	4.2	2,248	16	2,264
Cleveland-Lorain-Elyria, OH	170	7.6	199	8.9	3,894	46	3,940
Colorado Springs, CO	23	4.2	38	6.9	534	5	539
Columbia, SC	204	37.0	187	33.5	2,589	18	2,607
Columbus, OH	150	9.5	218	13.6	2,682	13	2,695
Dallas, TX	752	20.1	745	19.5	14,530	37	14,567
Dayton-Springfield, OH	46	4.9	100	10.6	1,201	17	1,218
Daytona Beach, FL	114	22.0	51	9.6	1,393	15	1,408
Denver, CO	230	10.5	261	11.8	6,319	22	6,341
Detroit, MI	579	13.0	483	10.8	9,176	74	9,250
El Paso, TX	79	11.4	92	13.0	1,350	10	1,360
Fort Lauderdale, FL	750	44.0	690	39.9	14,736	257	14,993
Fort Wayne, IN	31	6.1	18	3.5	382	3	385
Fort Worth-Arlington, TX	180	10.0	252	13.7	3,782	27	3,809
Fresno, CA	99	10.3	91	9.2	1,436	15	1,451
Gary, IN	62	9.7	45	7.0	887	6	893
Grand Rapids-Muskegon-Holland, MI	52	4.7	49	4.4	903	5	908
Greensboro/Winstn-Salem/H.Pt., NC	119	9.3	150	11.6	2,056	21	2,077
Greenville-Spartanburg-Andersn, SC	76	7.7	118	11.9	1,798	7	1,805
Harrisburg-Lebanon-Carlisle, PA	64	10.1	94	14.7	1,286	11	1,297
Hartford, CT Necma	199	17.0	285	24.2	4,624	47	4,671
Honolulu, HI	86	9.6	84	9.3	2,013	14	2,027
Houston, TX	979	22.2	1,324	29.4	22,014	166	22,180
Indianapolis, IN	275	16.6	263	15.7	3,575	24	3,599
Jacksonville, FL	271	23.5	283	24.0	5,255	73	5,328
Jersey City, NJ	199	32.6	172	28.3	7,096	121	7,217
Kansas City, MO-KS	125	6.8	138	7.5	4,333	13	4,346
Knoxville, TN	46	6.5	56	7.9	858	7	865
Lakeland-Winter Haven, FL	88	17.6	115	22.5	1,529	19	1,548
Las Vegas, NV-AZ	290	16.9	258	14.5	4,346	27	4,373
Little Rock-N. Little Rock, AR	89	15.0	53	8.8	1,260	14	1,274
Los Angeles-Long Beach, CA	1,549	15.9	2,558	25.9	47,136	243	47,379
Louisiville, KY-IN	137	13.2	110	10.5	2,025	19	2,044
McAllen-Edinburg-Mission, TX	42	6.8	46	7.2	501	11	512
Melbourne-Titusvlle-Palm Bay, FL	75	15.1	76	15.0	1,435	11	1,446
Memphis, TN-AR-MS	399	34.5	362	31.0	4,168	19	4,187
Miami, FL	1,139	49.2	1,072	45.8	27,023	502	27,525
Middlesex-Somerset-Hunterdon, NJ	140	11.6	118	9.7	3,541	73	3,614
Milwaukee-Waukesha, WI	113	7.5	103	6.8	2,284	19	2,303
Minneapolis-St. Paul, MN-WI	144	4.7	156	5.1	3,757	21	3,778
Mobile, AL	83	15.2	90	16.3	1,448	18	1,466
Monmouth-Ocean, NJ	100	8.6	84	7.1	3,127	64	3,191
Nashville, TN	196	15.4	271	21.0	3,353	17	3,370
Nassau-Suffolk, NJ	259	9.3	258	9.2	7,370	115	7,485

adolescents. (See Table 3.5.) The remaining 9,348 cases (representing 1% of the cumulative total) were children under the age of thirteen. According to the CDC, which has distinct case definitions for the two age groups, as of December 2003 more people between the ages of thirty-five and forty-four were living with either HIV or full-blown AIDS (168,322; 41.5% of all cases) than in any other age category. (See Table 3.6 and Table 3.7.)

Cumulatively, the total number of AIDS cases that were reported in adults and adolescents in 2003 occurred predominantly in males (729,478 cases). (See

TABLE 3.4

Reported AIDS cases and annual rates, by metropolitan area of residence and age category, cumulative through 2003 [CONTINUED]

	2002		2003		Cumulative through 2003		
					Adults or	Children	
Area of residence	No.	Rate	No.	Rate	adolescents	(<13 years)	Total
N Havn-Brpt-Dnbry-Wtrbry, CT Necma	358	20.7	396	22.7	7,535	125	7,660
New Orleans, LA	521	39.0	438	32.7	8,125	71	8,196
New York, NY	5,649	60.1	5,580	59.2	135,086	2,092	137,178
Newark, NJ	569	27.6	534	25.8	18,519	329	18,848
Norfolk-VA Beach-Newport News, VA	289	18.0	158	9.7	4,494	63	4,557
Oakland, CA	277	11.3	380	15.4	8,913	47	8,960
Oklahoma City, OK	107	9.7	100	8.9	2,097	7	2,104
Omaha, NE-IA	51	7.0	42	5.7	902	3	905
Orange County, CA	228	7.8	251	8.5	6,335	39	6,374
Orlando, FL	528	30.1	487	27.0	7,434	85	7,519
Philadelphia, PA-NJ	1,417	27.6	1,288	24.9	22,737	281	23,018
Phoenix-Mesa, AZ	512	14.7	421	11.7	6,557	28	6,585
Pittsburgh, PA	141	6.0	244	10.4	2,874	19	2,893
Portland-Vancouver, OR-WA	224	11.2	181	8.9	4,494	9	4,503
Providence-Warwick, RI Necma	100	10.2	92	9.3	2,191	23	2,214
Raleigh-Durham-Chapel Hill, NC	214	16.9	205	15.8	2,565	23	2,588
Richmond-Petersburg, VA	102	10.0	135	13.1	2,946	32	2,978
Riverside-San Bernardino, CA	282	8.1	472	13.0	7,933	58	7,991
Rochester, NY	191	17.4	138	12.5	2,786	13	2,799
Sacramento, CA	103	5.9	133	7.4	3,542	24	3,566
St. Louis, MO-IL	218	8.3	224	8.5	5,395	41	5,436
Salt Lake City-Ogden, UT	52	3.8	60	4.3	1,868	14	1,882
San Antonio, TX	200	12.0	166	9.8	4,484	28	4,512
San Diego, CA	467	16.1	516	17.6	11,945	58	12,003
San Francisco, CA	546	31.9	767	45.2	29,609	46	29,655
San Jose, CA	118	7.0	113	6.7	3,466	15	3,481
San Juan-Bayamon, PR	705	35.4	678	33.9	17,497	247	17,744
Sarasota-Bradenton, FL	105	16.9	123	19.4	1,801	25	1,826
Scranton—Wilkes-Barre—Hazleton, PA	24	3.9	33	5.4	497	5	502
Seattle-Bellevue-Everett, WA	316	12.8	380	15.3	7,673	19	7,692
Springfield, MA Necma	80	13.1	89	14.4	1,984	25	2,009
Stockton-Lodi, CA	80	13.0	80	12.6	935	13	948
Syracuse, NY	65	8.9	59	8.0	1,497	9	1,506
Tacoma, WA	32	4.4	34	4.6	963	9	972
Tampa-St Pete.-Clearwater, FL	504	20.3	557	22.0	9,933	105	10,038
Toledo, OH	56	9.0	36	5.8	701	12	713
Tucson, AZ	68	7.7	128	14.3	1,834	10	1,844
Tulsa, OK	49	6.0	66	8.0	1,312	10	1,322
Vallejo-Fairfield-Napa, CA	52	9.6	66	12.1	1,551	11	1,562
Ventura, CA	38	4.9	32	4.0	913	3	916
Washington, DC-MD-VA-WV	1,832	35.6	1,743	33.3	28,096	304	28,400
West Palm Beach-Boca Raton, FL	571	48.1	446	36.7	8,889	221	9,110
Wichita, KS	21	3.8	41	7.4	809	2	811
Wilmington-Newark, DE-MD	154	25.6	170	28.0	2,556	18	2,574
Youngstown-Warren, OH	24	4.1	25	4.3	444	0	444
Metropolitan areas with 500,000 or more population	35,728	19.2	36,548	19.4	749,638	7,950	757,588
Metropolitan areas with 50,000 to 499,999 population	4,337	8.9	4,608	9.4	83,394	832	84,226
Nonmetropolitan	3,220	5.7	3,414	6.0	54,828	515	55,343
Total*	**43,471**	**14.9**	**44,769**	**15.2**	**891,605**	**9,325**	**900,930**

Note: Includes persons from 50 states, the District of Columbia, and Puerto Rico, because of the lack of census information for the U.S. dependencies, possessions, and associated nations.

*Includes persons whose county of residence is unknown.

SOURCE: "Table 15. Reported AIDS Cases and Annual Rates (per 100,000 Population), by Metropolitan Area of Residence and Age Category, Cumulative through 2003—United States," in *HIV/AIDS Surveillance Report: Cases of HIV Infection and AIDS in the United States, 2003*, vol. 15, Centers for Disease Control and Prevention, 2004, http://www.cdc.gov/hiv/stats/2003SurveillanceReport.pdf (accessed July 18, 2005)

Table 3.5.) Adult and adolescent females accounted for 163,396 cumulative cases (18.6% of the total). (See Table 3.5.)

Race or Ethnicity and AIDS

The changing racial/ethnic profile characteristics of Americans with AIDS from 1993 through 2001 reflect a shift in the population at risk for HIV/AIDS. In 1993 there were 60,587 cases reported among African-Americans. By 2000 the number of cases had reached 135,562. (See Table 3.7.) The number of cases among African-Americans has grown steadily since (146,057 in 2001, 156,771 in 2002, and 167,938 in 2003). The corresponding case figures for non-Hispanic whites are 80,185

TABLE 3.5

Reported AIDS cases, by age category, transmission category, and sex, cumulative through 2003

	Males				Females				Total			
	2003		Cumulative through 2003[a]		2003		Cumulative through 2003[a]		2003		Cumulative through 2003[a]	
Transmission category	No.	%	No.	%	No.	%	No.	%	No.	%	No.	%
Adult or adolescent												
Male-to-male sexual contact	15,859	48	401,392	55	—	—	—	—	15,859	35	401,392	45
Injection drug use	4,866	15	156,575	21	2,262	20	61,621	38	7,128	16	218,196	24
Male-to-male sexual contact and injection drug use	1,695	5	57,998	8	—	—	—	—	1,695	4	57,998	6
Hemophilia/coagulation disorder	74	0	5,130	1	11	0	318	0	85	0	5,448	1
Heterosexual contact	3,371	10	40,947	6	5,234	45	70,200	43	8,605	19	111,147	12
Sex with injection drug user	477	1	10,930	1	985	9	24,148	15	1,462	3	35,078	4
Sex with bisexual male	0	0	0	0	223	2	4,402	3	223	0	4,402	0
Sex with person with hemophilia	7	0	80	0	16	0	465	0	23	0	545	0
Sex with HIV-infected transfusion recipient	24	0	505	0	37	0	705	0	61	0	1,210	0
Sex with HIV-infected person, risk factor not specified	2,863	9	29,432	4	3,973	34	40,480	25	6,836	15	69,912	8
Receipt of blood transfusion, blood components, or tissue[b]	111	0	5,219	1	108	1	4,076	2	219	0	9,295	1
Other/risk factor not reported or identified[c]	7,274	22	62,217	9	3,946	34	27,181	17	11,220	25	89,399	10
Subtotal	33,250	100	729,478	100	11,561	100	163,396	100	44,811	100	892,875	100
Child (<13 years at diagnosis)												
Hemophilia/coagulation disorder	0	0	227	5	0	0	7	0	0	0	234	3
Mother with the following risk factor for, or documented, HIV infection:	61	87	4,232	88	70	85	4,317	95	131	86	8,549	91
Injection drug use	6	9	1,643	34	11	13	1,645	36	17	11	3,288	35
Sex with injection drug user	8	11	784	16	6	7	741	16	14	9	1,525	16
Sex with bisexual male	0	0	95	2	2	2	102	2	2	1	197	2
Sex with person with hemophilia	1	1	21	0	0	0	15	0	1	1	36	0
Sex with HIV-infected transfusion recipient	0	0	11	0	0	0	16	0	0	0	27	0
Sex with HIV-infected person, risk factor not specified	18	26	705	15	18	22	737	16	36	24	1,442	15
Receipt of blood transfusion, blood components, or tissue	0	0	73	2	0	0	83	2	0	0	156	2
Has HIV infection, risk factor not specified	28	40	900	19	33	40	978	21	61	40	1,878	20
Receipt of blood transfusion, blood components, or tissue[b]	1	1	244	5	1	1	143	3	2	1	387	4
Other/risk factor not reported or identified[d]	8	11	80	2	11	13	98	2	19	13	178	2
Subtotal	70	100	4,783	100	82	100	4,565	100	152	100	9,348	100
Total	**33,320**	**100**	**734,261**	**100**	**11,643**	**100**	**167,961**	**100**	**44,963**	**100**	**902,223**	**100**

[a]Includes persons with a diagnosis of AIDS, reported from the beginning of the epidemic through 2003. Cumulative total includes 1 person of unknown sex.
[b]AIDS developed in 46 adults/adolescents and 3 children after they received blood that had tested negative for HIV antibodies. AIDS developed in 14 additional adults after they received tissue, organs, or artificial insemination from HIV-infected donors. Four of the 14 received tissue or organs from a donor who was negative for HIV antibody at the time of donation.
[c]Includes 36 adults/adolescents who were exposed to HIV-infected blood, body fluids, or concentrated virus in health care, laboratory, or household settings, as supported by seroconversion, epidemiologic, and/or laboratory evidence. One person was infected after intentional inoculation with HIV-infected blood. For an additional 361 persons who acquired HIV infection perinatally, AIDS was diagnosed after age 13. These 361 persons are tabulated under the adult/adolescent, not the pediatric, transmission category.
[d]Includes 5 children who were exposed to HIV-infected blood as supported by seroconversion, epidemiologic, and/or laboratory evidence: 1 child was infected after intentional inoculation with HIV-infected blood and 4 children were exposed to HIV-infected blood in a household setting. Of the 178 children, 23 had sexual contact with an adult with or at high risk for HIV infection.

SOURCE: "Table 17. Reported AIDS Cases, by Age Category, Transmission Category, and Sex, Cumulative through 2003—United States," in *HIV/AIDS Surveillance Report: Cases of HIV Infection and AIDS in the United States, 2003*, vol. 15, Centers for Disease Control and Prevention, 2004, http://www.cdc.gov/hiv/stats/2003SurveillanceReport.pdf (accessed July 18, 2005)

in 1993, 113,617 in 2000, 120,186 in 2001, 127,257 in 2002, and 134,678 in 2003. The number of AIDS cases among African-Americans has exceeded those among whites from 1998 through 2003.

In 1999 African-Americans accounted for 40.6% of people estimated to be living with HIV/AIDS. This figure rose to 47.7% in 2001 through 2003. In contrast, the proportion of non-Hispanic whites living with HIV/AIDS

TABLE 3.6

Estimated numbers of persons living with AIDS, by year and selected characteristics, 1999–2003

	1999	2000	2001	2002	2003
Age as of end of year (years)					
<13	3,034	2,843	2,605	2,335	1,998
13–14	440	517	645	728	768
15–24	4,719	4,991	5,229	5,668	6,313
25–34	60,184	56,686	53,687	51,410	49,906
35–44	141,295	151,180	158,173	163,732	168,322
45–54	77,216	89,461	102,252	115,613	129,311
55–64	19,258	22,922	27,197	32,703	38,997
≥65	5,058	6,132	7,251	8,583	10,310
Race/ethnicity					
White, not Hispanic	119,674	126,162	132,258	139,089	146,544
Black, not Hispanic	126,044	137,524	148,469	160,022	172,278
Hispanic	61,194	66,266	71,034	75,782	80,623
Asian/Pacific Islander	2,484	2,755	3,056	3,414	3,826
American Indian/Alaska Native	1,047	1,166	1,262	1,380	1,498
Transmission category					
Male adult or adolescent					
Male-to-male sexual contact	140,216	150,172	160,076	171,035	182,989
Injection drug use	58,006	61,249	63,723	66,003	68,191
Male-to-male sexual contact and injection drug use	21,667	22,403	23,033	23,690	24,334
Heterosexual contact	20,595	23,478	26,471	29,835	33,324
Other[a]	3,807	3,922	4,062	4,204	4,345
Subtotal	244,291	261,223	277,366	294,767	313,183
Female adult or adolescent					
Injection drug use	25,744	27,317	28,602	29,670	30,710
Heterosexual contact	35,603	40,422	45,097	50,142	55,685
Other[a]	1,746	1,908	2,067	2,239	2,420
Subtotal	63,093	69,647	75,765	82,052	88,815
Child (<13 years at diagnosis)					
Perinatal	3,672	3,714	3,763	3,808	3,788
Other[b]	148	145	145	143	139
Subtotal	3,820	3,860	3,908	3,951	3,927
Region of residence					
Northeast	92,741	99,964	105,970	111,506	116,827
Midwest	31,016	33,470	35,725	38,513	41,668
South	115,991	125,396	135,465	146,421	158,962
West	62,300	66,280	69,931	74,253	78,333
U.S. dependencies, possessions, and associated nations	9,157	9,621	9,949	10,077	10,136
Total[c]	**311,205**	**334,731**	**357,040**	**380,771**	**405,926**

Note: These numbers do not represent reported case counts. Rather, these numbers are point estimates, which result from adjustments of reported case counts. The reported case counts are adjusted for reporting delays and for redistribution of cases in persons initially reported without an identified risk factor. The estimates do not include adjustment for incomplete reporting.

[a]Includes hemophilia, blood transfusion, perinatal, and risk factor not reported or not identified.
[b]Includes hemophilia, blood transfusion, and risk factor not reported or not identified.
[c]Includes persons of unknown race or multiple races and persons of unknown sex. Because column totals were calculated independently of the values for the subpopulations, the values in each column may not sum to the column total.

SOURCE: "Table 10. Estimated Numbers of Persons Living with AIDS, by Year and Selected Characteristics, 1999–2003—United States," in *HIV/AIDS Surveillance Report: Cases of HIV Infection and AIDS in the United States, 2003*, vol. 15, Centers for Disease Control and Prevention, 2004, http://www.cdc.gov/hiv/stats/2003SurveillanceReport.pdf (accessed July 18, 2005)

went from 38.5% (1999) to 39.2% (2001), 38.7% (2002), and 38.3% (2003).

In 2003 Hispanics accounted for 9,133 new reported AIDS cases. Corresponding figures for whites and African-Americans were 13,612 and 21,064, respectively. The total number of male and female adult and adolescent reported AIDS cases in Asian-Americans/Pacific Islanders (558) and Native Americans/Alaska Natives (220) were the lowest of all racial/ ethnic groups in the United States. (See Table 3.8 and Table 3.9.)

In 2003 the total (male and female) reported AIDS incidence rate per one hundred thousand adults and adolescents among African-Americans (75.2) was more than ten times higher than that among non-Hispanic white Americans (7.2), more than seven times than that of Native Americans/Alaska Natives (10.4), and almost three times that of Hispanics (26.8). Rates were lowest

TABLE 3.7

Estimated numbers of persons living with HIV/AIDS by year, 2000–03

	2000	2001	2002	2003
Age as of end of year (years)				
<13	2,898	2,867	2,796	2,614
13–14	336	442	519	618
15–24	11,297	11,931	12,409	13,134
25–34	67,688	66,711	66,416	66,446
35–44	124,116	132,137	139,133	145,288
45–54	60,616	70,407	80,757	91,567
55–64	14,579	17,314	20,988	25,237
≥65	4,002	4,840	5,687	6,710
Race/ethnicity				
White, not Hispanic	113,617	120,186	127,257	134,678
Black, not Hispanic	135,562	146,057	156,771	167,938
Hispanic	31,950	35,508	39,358	43,241
Asian/Pacific Islander	1,034	1,171	1,344	1,595
American Indian/Alaska Native	1,508	1,606	1,737	1,873
Transmission category				
Male adult or adolescent				
Male-to-male sexual contact	128,956	138,629	149,336	160,433
Injection drug use	36,526	38,098	39,630	41,207
Male-to-male sexual contact and injection drug use	19,097	19,642	20,175	20,773
Heterosexual contact	25,262	28,115	31,042	34,124
Other[a]	2,817	2,891	2,972	3,071
Subtotal	212,658	227,375	243,154	259,609
Female adult or adolescent				
Injection drug use	19,789	20,650	21,381	22,173
Heterosexual contact	47,963	53,245	58,547	63,981
Other[a]	1,450	1,547	1,660	1,787
Subtotal	69,202	75,442	81,588	87,940
Child (<13 years at diagnosis)				
Perinatal	3,260	3,434	3,593	3,720
Other[b]	406	393	367	342
Subtotal	3,666	3,827	3,960	4,062
Total[c]	**285,531**	**306,649**	**328,705**	**351,614**

Note: These numbers do not represent reported case counts. Rather, these numbers are point estimates, which result from adjustments of reported case counts. The reported case counts are adjusted for reporting delays and for redistribution of cases in persons initially reported without an identified risk factor. The estimates do not include adjustment for incomplete reporting.

Data include persons with a diagnosis of HIV infection. This includes persons with a diagnosis of HIV only, a diagnosis of HIV infection and a later AIDS diagnosis, and concurrent diagnoses of HIV infection and AIDS.

Since 1999, the following 33 areas have had laws or regulations requiring confidential name-based HIV infection reporting: Alabama, Alaska, Arizona, Arkansas, Colorado, Florida, Idaho, Indiana, Iowa, Kansas, Louisiana, Michigan, Minnesota, Mississippi, Missouri, Nebraska, Nevada, New Jersey, New Mexico, North Carolina, North Dakota, Ohio, Oklahoma, South Carolina, South Dakota, Tennessee, Texas, Utah, Virginia, West Virginia, Wisconsin, Wyoming, and the U.S. Virgin Islands. Since July 1997, Florida has had confidential name-based HIV infection reporting only for new diagnoses.

[a]Includes hemophilia, blood transfusion, perinatal, and risk factor not reported or not identified.

[b]Includes hemophilia, blood transfusion, and risk factor not reported or not identified.

[c]Includes persons of unknown race or multiple races and persons of unknown sex. Because column totals were calculated independently of the values for the subpopulations, the values in each column may not sum to the column total.

SOURCE: "Table 8. Estimated Numbers of Persons Living with HIV/AIDS, by Year and Selected Characteristics, 2000–2003—33 Areas with Confidential Name-Based HIV Infection Reporting," in *HIV/AIDS Surveillance Report: Cases of HIV Infection and AIDS in the United States, 2003*, vol. 15, Centers for Disease Control and Prevention, 2004, http://www.cdc.gov/hiv/stats/2003SurveillanceReport.pdf (accessed July 18, 2005)

among Asian-Americans/Pacific Islanders (4.8). (See Table 3.10.)

The racial and ethnic difference is particularly alarming among children under the age of thirteen. As shown in Table 3.10, in 2003 the rate of HIV per one hundred thousand population for African-American children (0.5) was five times the rate for Hispanic children (0.1). The other categories were negligible.

The racial disparity is also reflected in the acquisition of HIV/AIDS by infants born to HIV-infected mothers. In the years 2000 through 2003 the number of reported cases of HIV/AIDS among African-American infants has been a minimum of four times greater than the reported cases for non-Hispanic whites and Hispanic infants born to HIV-infected mothers. (See Table 3.11.)

HOW HIV IS TRANSMITTED

HIV can be transmitted by sexual contact with an infected person; by needle sharing among infected

TABLE 3.8

Reported AIDS cases for female adults and adolescents, by transmission category and race/ethnicity, cumulative through 2003

Transmission category	White, not Hispanic 2003 No.	%	Cumulative through 2003* No.	%	Black, not Hispanic 2003 No.	%	Cumulative through 2003* No.	%	Hispanic 2003 No.	%	Cumulative through 2003* No.	%
Injection drug use	557	29	13,695	41	1,277	17	35,767	37	385	18	11,695	37
Hemophilia/coagulation disorder	3	0	117	0	5	0	128	0	3	0	60	0
Heterosexual contact:	809	42	13,877	41	3,253	44	40,193	42	1,055	50	15,294	48
Sex with injection drug user	220	12	5,293	16	525	7	12,526	13	218	10	6,103	19
Sex with bisexual male	47	2	1,701	5	118	2	1,885	2	54	3	701	2
Sex with person with hemophilia	12	1	314	1	3	0	103	0	1	0	42	0
Sex with HIV-infected transfusion recipient	4	0	334	1	25	0	230	0	7	0	114	0
Sex with HIV-infected person, risk factor not specified	526	28	6,235	19	2,582	35	25,449	26	775	37	8,334	26
Receipt of blood transfusion, blood components, or tissue	18	1	1,868	6	60	1	1,477	2	25	1	604	2
Other/risk factor not reported or identified	522	27	4,127	12	2,734	37	18,796	20	630	30	3,901	
Total	**1,909**	**100**	**33,684**	**100**	**7,329**	**100**	**96,361**	**100**	**2,098**	**100**	**31,554**	**100**

Transmission category	Islander Asian/Pacific 2003 No.	%	Cumulative through 2003* No.	%	American Indian/Alaska Native 2003 No.	%	Cumulative through 2003* No.	%	Totals 2003 No.	%	Cumulative through 2003* No.	%
Injection drug use	6	6	121	13	23	39	242	43	2,262	20	61,621	38
Hemophilia/coagulation disorder	0	0	8	1	0	0	3	1	11	0	318	0
Heterosexual contact:	56	55	459	51	22	37	228	41	5,234	45	70,200	43
Sex with injection drug user	11	11	104	12	4	7	92	16	985	9	24,148	15
Sex with bisexual male	3	3	78	9	1	2	29	5	223	2	4,402	3
Sex with person with hemophilia	0	0	4	0	0	0	2	0	16	0	465	0
Sex with HIV-infected transfusion recipient	1	1	20	2	0	0	3	1	37	0	705	0
Sex with HIV-infected person, risk factor not specified	41	40	253	28	17	29	102	18	3,973	34	40,480	25
Receipt of blood transfusion, blood components, or tissue	4	4	101	11	1	2	15	3	108	1	4,076	2
Other/risk factor not reported or identified	36	35	212	24	13	22	70	13	3,946	34	27,181	17
Total	**102**	**100**	**901**	**100**	**59**	**100**	**558**	**100**	**11,561**	**100**	**163,396**	**100**

*Includes persons with a diagnosis of AIDS, reported from the beginning of the epidemic through 2003. Cumulative total includes 338 females of unknown race or multiple races.

SOURCE: "Table 21. Reported AIDS Cases for Female Adults and Adolescents, by Transmission Category and Race/Ethnicity, Cumulative through 2003—United States," in *HIV/AIDS Surveillance Report: Cases of HIV Infection and AIDS in the United States, 2003*, vol. 15, Centers for Disease Control and Prevention, 2004, http://www.cdc.gov/hiv/stats/2003SurveillanceReport.pdf (accessed July 18, 2005)

intravenous drug users; through the receipt of infected blood, blood products, or tissue; and directly from an infected mother to her infant during pregnancy, delivery, or breastfeeding.

In the United States MTM remain the majority of HIV carriers, although prevalence among heterosexuals is on the rise. In 1987, 70% of adult and adolescent males with AIDS had a single risk factor of a history of high-risk sexual activity. The proportion of affected MTM has dropped to 45% (2001 through 2003). Adult and adolescent males with a history of intravenous drug use as their only risk factor made up 14% of all cases in 1987. This proportion has changed only marginally in the intervening years, remaining relatively stable at 15% in 2003. (See Table 3.9.)

The proportion of adult and adolescent females with AIDS whose only risk factor was intravenous drug use has dropped from 50% in 1987 to 39% in 2001. Adult and adolescent females with a history of heterosexual contact as their only risk factor made up 38% of all female cases in 1997. By 2001 that proportion increased to 41%, and through 2003 has increased to 45%. (See Table 3.8.) Researchers suggest that one reason for steadily increasing HIV infection and AIDS among heterosexuals is that an increased proportion report multiple sex partners, which is a risk factor for HIV infection.

Undetermined Risk

In 2003 there were 11,220 adult and adolescent (both male and female) cases of AIDS with an undetermined

TABLE 3.9

Reported AIDS cases for male adults and adolescents, by transmission category and race/ethnicity, cumulative through 2003

Transmission category	White, not Hispanic 2003 No.	%	Cumulative through 2003* No.	%	Black, not Hispanic 2003 No.	%	Cumulative through 2003* No.	%	Hispanic 2003 No.	%	Cumulative through 2003* No.	%
Male-to-male sexual contact	7,679	66	244,758	73	4,699	34	93,413	37	3,054	43	57,128	43
Injection drug use	1,051	9	31,164	9	2,454	18	80,282	32	1,290	18	44,277	33
Male-to-male sexual contact and injection drug use	793	7	28,795	9	548	4	19,182	8	311	4	9,313	7
Hemophilia/coagulation disorder	56	0	3,964	1	6	0	599	0	9	0	453	0
Heterosexual contact:	454	4	7,010	2	2,047	15	24,428	10	799	11	9,021	7
Sex with injection drug user	76	1	2,221	1	253	2	6,410	3	141	2	2,195	2
Sex with person with hemophilia	4	0	38	0	2	0	29	0	0	0	11	0
Sex with HIV-infected transfusion recipient	4	0	177	0	11	0	205	0	7	0	109	0
Sex with HIV-infected person, risk factor not specified	370	3	4,574	1	1,781	13	17,784	7	651	9	6,706	5
Receipt of blood transfusion, blood components, or tissue	30	0	3,227	1	49	0	1,205	0	28	0	646	0
Other/risk factor not reported or identified	1,640	14	14,519	4	3,932	29	33,905	13	1,544	22	12,659	9
Total	**11,703**	**100**	**333,437**	**100**	**13,735**	**100**	**253,014**	**100**	**7,035**	**100**	**133,497**	**100**

Transmission category	Asian/Pacific Islander 2003 No.	%	Cumulative through 2003* No.	%	American Indian/Alaska Native 2003 No.	%	Cumulative through 2003* No.	%	Total 2003 No.	%	Cumulative through 2003* No.	%
Male-to-male sexual contact	254	56	4,084	69	93	58	1,299	56	15,859	48	401,392	55
Injection drug use	26	6	292	5	22	14	370	16	4,866	15	156,575	21
Male-to-male sexual contact and injection drug use	19	4	227	4	15	9	392	17	1,695	5	57,998	8
Hemophilia/coagulation disorder	2	0	72	1	1	1	32	1	74	0	5,130	1
Heterosexual contact:	42	9	305	5	11	7	92	4	3,371	10	40,947	6
Sex with injection drug user	3	1	55	1	2	1	28	1	477	1	10,930	1
Sex with person with hemophilia	0	0	1	0	0	0	0	0	7	0	80	0
Sex with HIV-infected transfusion recipient	1	0	8	0	1	1	3	0	24	0	505	0
Sex with HIV-infected person, risk factor not specified	38	8	241	4	8	5	61	3	2,863	9	29,432	4
Receipt of blood transfusion, blood components, or tissue	3	1	118	2	0	0	9	0	111	0	5,219	1
Other/risk factor not reported or identified	110	24	792	13	19	12	130	6	7,274	22	62,217	9
Total	**456**	**100**	**5,890**	**100**	**161**	**100**	**2,324**	**100**	**33,250**	**100**	**729,478**	**100**

*Includes persons with a diagnosis of AIDS, reported from the beginning of the epidemic through 2003. Cumulative total includes 1,316 males of unknown race or multiple races.

SOURCE: "Table 19. Reported AIDS Cases for Males and Adolescents, by Transmission Category and Race/Ethnicity, Cumulative through 2003—United States," in *HIV/AIDS Surveillance Report: Cases of HIV Infection and AIDS in the United States, 2003*, vol. 15, Centers for Disease Control and Prevention, 2004, http://www.cdc.gov/hiv/stats/2003SurveillanceReport.pdf (accessed July 18, 2005)

risk. (See Table 3.5.) That is, there was no reported history of exposure to HIV through any of the routes listed in the exposure categories. These include people currently being investigated by local health departments, people whose exposure history was incomplete at the time of their death, those who refused to be interviewed or whose cases were not followed up, and those who were interviewed but no follow-up occurred. When an exposure mode is identified during follow-up, patients are reclassified into the appropriate exposure category.

MORTALITY FROM AIDS

By 1999 the average life expectancy for Americans had risen to an all-time high of 76.7 years. This figure would have been higher, according to the CDC, were it not for heart diseases (the leading cause of death for all age categories), malignant neoplasms (the leading cause of death for those ages forty-five to sixty-four), and accidents (the leading cause of death for those ages fifteen to forty-four). AIDS is also among the top ten leading causes of death among the latter age group.

TABLE 3.10

Estimated number of cases and rates of AIDS, by race/ethnicity, age category, and sex, 2003

| Race/ethnicity | Adults or adolescents | | | | | | Children (<13 years) | | Total | |
| | Males | | Females | | Total | | | | | |
	No.	Rate	No.	Rate	No.	Rate	No.	Rate	No.	Rate
White, not Hispanic	10,450	12.8	1,725	2.0	12,175	7.2	9	0.0	12,184	6.1
Black, not Hispanic	13,624	103.8	7,551	50.2	21,174	75.2	40	0.5	21,214	58.2
Hispanic	6,087	40.3	1,744	12.4	7,831	26.8	7	0.1	7,839	20.0
Asian/Pacific Islander	408	8.3	86	1.6	494	4.8	0	0	494	4.0
American Indian/Alaska Native	150	16.2	46	4.8	196	10.4	0	0	196	8.1
Total*	**30,851**	**26.6**	**11,211**	**9.2**	**42,062**	**17.7**	**58**	**0.1**	**42,120**	**14.5**

Note: These numbers do not represent reported case counts. Rather, these numbers are point estimates, which result from adjustments of reported case counts. The reported case counts are adjusted for reporting delays. The estimates do not include adjustment for incomplete reporting.

Data exclude cases from the U.S. dependencies, possessions, and associated nations, as well as cases in persons whose state or area of residence is unknown, because of the lack of census information by race and age categories for these areas.

*Includes persons of unknown race or multiple races. Total includes 193 persons of unknown race or multiple races. Because column totals were calculated independently of the values for the subpopulations, the values in each column may not sum to the column total.

SOURCE: "Table 5. Estimated Numbers of Cases and Rates (per 100,000 Population) of AIDS, by Race/Ethnicity, Age Category, and Sex, 2003—50 States and the District of Columbia," in *HIV/AIDS Surveillance Report: Cases of HIV Infection and AIDS in the United States, 2003*, vol. 15, Centers for Disease Control and Prevention, 2004, http://www.cdc.gov/hiv/stats/2003SurveillanceReport.pdf (accessed July 18, 2005)

According to CDC statistics compiled in 2003, since 1999 AIDS has claimed the lives of 368,643 Americans ages fifteen to forty-four, representing 70% of the total numbers of deaths (524,060). (See Table 3.2.)

Nearly 100% of AIDS patients die within seven years of the initial diagnosis of the late stage of HIV infection. Some deaths are not reported to the CDC or are reported as deaths from other causes. So the reported case-fatality rate (the number of deaths from a disease divided by the number of cases of that disease) is surely an underestimate. The case-fatality rate is frequently used as a measure of the severity of a disease and to estimate the probability of death among diagnosed cases.

The number of deaths due to AIDS peaked at 51,670 in 1995. Since then the number of deaths has been dropping. In 2003 the disease killed 18,017 Americans. Fewer people are dying from AIDS because of more effective treatment. As fewer people become infected with HIV, the death rate in subsequent years will drop proportionally. The statistics for children under the age of thirteen at the time of diagnosis, however, remain grim—half die before their first birthday, while the other half do not live to adolescence.

According to 2001 CDC data (the latest available as of this writing), 70% (328,588) of the males and females who have died from AIDS since the epidemic began were aged twenty-five to forty-four. In that age group, 49,839 (11%) were female and 278,749 (60%) were male. White and black males made up the largest group of cumulative deaths (139,152 and 87,774, respectively), with Hispanic males (48,902) and black females (28,918) ranking third and fourth.

TABLE 3.11

Reported cases of HIV/AIDS in infants born to HIV-infected mothers, by selected characteristics, 2000–03

	Year of report			
	2000	**2001**	**2002**	**2003**
Child's race/ethnicity				
White, not Hispanic	14	20	22	15
Black, not Hispanic	90	91	68	62
Hispanic	17	15	18	8
Asian/Pacific Islander	1	1	1	1
American Indian/Alaska Native	0	0	1	1
Perinatal transmission category				
Mother with, or at risk for, HIV infection:				
Injection drug use	32	26	10	7
Sex with injection drug user	12	11	11	6
Sex with bisexual male	2	5	2	5
Sex with person with hemophilia	1	1	0	1
Sex with HIV-infected transfusion recipient	0	0	0	0
Sex with HIV-infected person, risk not specified	44	47	39	38
Receipt of blood transfusion, blood components, or tissue	0	3	1	0
Has HIV infection, risk not specified	31	34	48	33
Child's diagnosis status[a]				
HIV infection	95	91	77	75
AIDS	27	36	34	15
Total[b]	**122**	**127**	**111**	**90**

Note: Since 1994, the following 25 states have had laws and regulations requiring confidential name-based HIV infection reporting: Alabama, Arizona, Arkansas, Colorado, Idaho, Indiana, Louisiana, Michigan, Minnesota, Mississippi, Missouri, Nevada, New Jersey, North Carolina, North Dakota, Ohio, Oklahoma, South Carolina, South Dakota, Tennessee, Utah, Virginia, West Virginia, Wisconsin, and Wyoming.
Data include children with a diagnosis of HIV infection. This includes children with a diagnosis of HIV infection only, a diagnosis of HIV infection and a later AIDS diagnosis, and concurrent diagnoses of HIV infection and AIDS.
[a]Status in the surveillance system as of June 2004.
[b]Includes children of unknown or multiple race.

SOURCE: "Table 23. Reported Cases of HIV/AIDS in Infants Born to HIV-Infected Mothers, by Year of Report and Selected Characteristics, 1994–2003—25 States with Confidential Name-Based HIV Infection Reporting," in *HIV/AIDS Surveillance Report: Cases of HIV Infection and AIDS in the United States, 2003*, vol. 15, Centers for Disease Control and Prevention, 2004, http://www.cdc.gov/hiv/stats/2003SurveillanceReport.pdf (accessed July 18, 2005)

CHAPTER 4
POPULATIONS AT RISK

This chapter examines the prevalence rates of HIV infection—that is, the number of people who have the disease in a specified time period versus the total number of people in the population being examined. The prevalence rates are based on surveys of selected segments of the general population and the prevalence rates of people in high-risk groups. These are not absolute numbers. The actual number of cases of HIV infection is likely to be higher than those reported here, since reporting is not universal and, as of June 2005, only thirty-eight U.S. states and the U.S. territories of Guam and the Virgin Islands subscribe to confidential reporting practices. But information on prevalence rates serves as a road map revealing trends and geographical or societal areas of special concern.

INCREASE IN AIDS AMONG HETEROSEXUALS

The increase in the number and proportion of HIV/AIDS cases among heterosexuals signals a major shift in the patterns of the epidemic. In 1997 the Centers for Disease Control and Prevention (CDC) reported that people diagnosed with AIDS who acquired HIV through heterosexual transmission accounted for the largest proportional increase of all cases in the previous year. During 2003, 44,963 new cases of AIDS among adults and adolescents were reported to the CDC. Nineteen percent of these new cases (8,605) were people who reported that their only exposure was through heterosexual contact. (See Table 3.5 in Chapter 3.) In comparison, in 1985 less than 2% of all AIDS cases were attributable to heterosexual transmission.

Between 1997 and 2000 the number of new AIDS cases dropped significantly, and the proportions of those infected in each exposure category also changed. Cases attributed to male-to-male sexual contact (MTM) represented 35% of all cases in 1997 and 1998, dropping to 34% in 1999, 32% in 2000, and 31% in 2001. In 2003 the MTM rate was again 35%. In spite of the decline from the late 1990s, MTM continued to represent the largest

proportion (46% in both 2000 and 2001, and 45% in 2003) of cumulative AIDS cases since 1981. Among women, intravenous drug use decreased from 32% of all exposures in 1997 to 25% in 2000 and 20% in both 2001 and 2003. The overall incidence of AIDS based on heterosexual exposure has steadily increased, from 13% in 1997 to 16% in both 2000 and 2001 and then up to 19% in 2003. The proportion of women who contracted AIDS through heterosexual contact remained relatively constant at 38% in 2002 and 37% in 2001. However, in 2003 the proportion increased to 45%.

Risks of Heterosexual Contact

Data reported in 2003 reveal that 15% of adult and adolescent AIDS cases attributed to heterosexual contact resulted from sexual contact with an HIV-infected partner of an unspecified risk category (6,836 out of 44,963). In 2001 the numbers were 5,181 out of 42,983 (12%) and in 2000 4,799 out of 41,960 (11%). The actual number of cases reported during 2003 represents an 8% increase from the number of cases reported during 2001, with the 2001 number representing a 7% increase from the number of cases reported during 2000. A smaller proportion of cases in 2003 (3%, representing 1,462 cases out of 44,963) was attributed to heterosexual contact with an intravenous drug user. The data from 2001 and 2000 were very similar (3.5%, representing 1,486 cases out of 42,983 in 2001, and 3.6%, representing 1,496 cases out of 41,960 in 2000).

During 2000 heterosexual transmission accounted for 2,448 new cases of HIV infection reported among women in the United States, most of whom were African-American (67%). In 2001 the number of cases rose to 3,071, with African-American women accounting for 65% of cases. In 2003 the number of cases rose again, to 5,234, with African-American women accounting for 44%. (See Table 3.8 in Chapter 3.)

TABLE 4.1

Reported HIV cases for male adults and adolescents, by transmission category and race/ethnicity, cumulative through 2003

Transmission category	White, not Hispanic				Black, not Hispanic				Hispanic			
	2003		Cumulative through 2003*		2003		Cumulative through 2003*		2003		Cumulative through 2003*	
	No.	%	No.	%	No.	%	No.	%	No.	%	No.	%
Male-to-male sexual contact	5,464	65	41,048	65	2,944	32	21,472	33	1,853	37	8,941	42
Injection drug use	578	7	4,969	8	1,009	11	10,658	16	945	19	3,815	18
Male-to-male sexual contact and injection drug use	387	5	4,606	7	192	2	3,011	5	139	3	838	4
Hemophilia/coagulation disorder	33	0	381	1	9	0	107	0	6	0	27	0
Heterosexual contact:	307	4	2,053	3	1,212	13	8,681	13	466	9	1,766	8
Sex with injection drug user	67	1	490	1	63	2	1,445	2	74	1	304	1
Sex with person with hemophilia	5	0	7	0	0	0	14	0	1	0	4	0
Sex with HIV-infected transfusion recipient	4	0	27	0	9	0	76	0	2	0	11	0
Sex with HIV-infected person, risk factor not specified	231	3	1,529	2	1,040	11	7,146	11	389	8	1,447	7
Receipt of blood transfusion, blood components, or tissue	13	0	216	0	8	0	204	0	3	0	46	0
Other/risk factor not reported or identified	1,572	19	9,676	15	3,708	41	21,183	32	1,618	32	5,968	28
Total	**8,354**	**100**	**62,949**	**100**	**9,082**	**100**	**65,316**	**100**	**5,030**	**100**	**21,401**	**100**

Transmission category	Asian/Pacific Islander				American Indian/Alaska Native				Total			
	2003		Cumulative through 2003*		2003		Cumulative through 2003*		2003		Cumulative through 2003*	
	No.	%	No.	%	No.	%	No.	%	No.	%	No.	%
Male-to-male sexual contact	118	59	493	54	49	53	428	55	10,466	46	72,745	48
Injection drug use	9	5	46	5	8	9	89	11	2,551	11	19,652	13
Male-to-male sexual contact and injection drug use	5	3	20	2	6	7	103	13	732	3	8,623	6
Hemophilia/coagulation disorder	0	0	2	0	0	0	0	0	48	0	520	0
Heterosexual contact:	7	4	57	6	8	9	51	7	2,009	9	12,669	8
Sex with injection drug user	1	1	8	1	1	1	16	2	307	1	2,272	1
Sex with person with hemophilia	0	0	0	0	0	0	0	0	6	0	25	0
Sex with HIV-infected transfusion recipient	0	0	2	0	0	0	0	0	15	0	116	0
Sex with HIV-infected person, risk factor not specified	6	3	47	5	7	8	35	4	1,681	7	10,256	7
Receipt of blood transfusion, blood components, or tissue	1	1	3	0	0	0	2	0	26	0	477	0
Other/risk factor not reported or identified	60	30	290	32	21	23	111	14	7,003	31	38,053	25
Total	**200**	**100**	**911**	**100**	**92**	**100**	**784**	**100**	**22,835**	**100**	**152,739**	**100**

Note: Includes only persons with HIV infection that has not progressed to AIDS. Since 2003, the following 41 areas have had laws or regulations requiring confidential name-based HIV infection reporting: Alabama, Alaska, Arizona, Arkansas, Colorado, Connecticut, Florida, Georgia, Idaho, Indiana, Iowa, Kansas, Louisiana, Michigan, Minnesota, Mississippi, Missouri, Nebraska, Nevada, New Jersey, New Mexico, New York, North Carolina, North Dakota, Ohio, Oklahoma, Pennsylvania, Puerto Rico, South Carolina, South Dakota, Tennessee, Texas, Utah, Virginia, West Virginia, Wisconsin, Wyoming, American Samoa, Guam, Northern Mariana Islands, and the U.S. Virgin Islands. Connecticut has confidential name-based HIV infection reporting only for pediatric cases. Florida (since July 1997) has had confidential name-based HIV infection reporting only for new diagnoses. Pennsylvania (October 2002) implemented confidential name-based HIV infection reporting only in areas outside the city of Philadelphia. Texas (February 1994 through December 1998) reported only pediatric HIV infection cases.
*Includes persons with a diagnosis of HIV infection (not AIDS), reported from the beginning of the epidemic through December 2003. Cumulative total includes 1,378 males of unknown race or multiple races.

SOURCE: "Table 20. Reported Cases of HIV Infection (Not AIDS) for Male Adults and Adolescents, by Transmission Category and Race/Ethnicity, Cumulative through 2003," in *HIV/AIDS Surveillance Report: Cases of HIV Infection and AIDS in the United States, 2003*, vol. 15, Centers for Disease Control and Prevention, 2004, http://www.cdc.gov/hiv/stats/2003SurveillanceReport.pdf (accessed July 18, 2005)

Among heterosexual men, 1,231 cases of HIV were reported in 2000, 1,466 in 2001, and 2,009 in 2003. In 2000, 73% of these men were African-American and 11% were Hispanic. In 2001 the number fell to 68% for African- Americans but rose to 16% for Hispanics. Finally, in 2003 the percentage of heterosexual transmission was 60% for African-Americans (1,212 cases out of 2,009) and 23% (466 cases out of 2,009) for Hispanics. (See Table 4.1.)

INTRAVENOUS DRUG USERS

The National Academy of Sciences (NAS) concluded in a 1995 report to Congress that "the HIV epidemic in this country is now clearly driven by infections occurring in the population of drug users, their sexual partners, and their offspring." During the 1990s the proportions of both HIV infection and AIDS deaths attributable to intravenous drug use (IDU) among adults and adolescents increased. In 1999 IDU was the exposure category for 32% of male and 47% of female AIDS deaths. To offset the rise in IDU-associated HIV infection and AIDS, the NAS urged members of Congress to adequately fund needle exchange programs. Since 1999 the percentage of HIV/AIDS cases attributable to IDU has been steadily decreasing. Of the 22,835 men and 11,561 women reported as HIV-infected during 2003, 11% of men (2,551 cases) and 20% (2,262 cases) of women reported IDU as the sole exposure category. (See Table 3.8 in Chapter 3 and Table 4.1.)

How HIV Is Transmitted through Drug Use

HIV can be transmitted through IDU when the blood of an HIV-infected drug user is transferred to a drug user who is not yet infected with HIV. This transfer occurs almost exclusively through the sharing of injecting equipment, primarily needles and syringes.

Blood makes it into the needle and syringe in two ways. The first occurs when blood is drawn from the syringe to verify that the needle is inside a vein, prior to the injection of the drug. The second occurs following the injection, when the syringe is refilled several times with blood from the vein to "wash out" any heroin, cocaine, or other drug left in the syringe after the first injection. Even the smallest amount of HIV-infected blood left in the syringe can cause the virus to be transmitted to the next user of the contaminated syringe and needle.

Among IDUs the risk of HIV infection increases in proportion to the duration of intravenous drug use. Put another way, the longer the drug use, the greater the risk of infection. Diseases such as hepatitis show this same pattern. Risk also increases with the frequency of needle sharing and intravenous drug use in a geographic area, such as a large city, where there is a high prevalence of HIV infection.

General Trends

Table 3.5 in Chapter 3 shows that, of the cumulative AIDS cases among adults and adolescents reported from 1981 through December 2003 (902,223), 218,196 were attributable to intravenous drug use (24%). Cumulatively, slightly more than 6% (57,998 cases) was attributable to MTM contact in conjunction with intravenous drug use, and an additional 4% (35,078 cases) was the result of heterosexual contact with an IDU.

HIV is also spread among non-IDUs who trade sex for drugs, especially "crack" cocaine, as well as the partners of these users. Those who trade sex for drugs often engage in unprotected sex and have multiple sex partners. People who exchange sex for drugs and have a sexually transmitted disease (STD) that causes ulcers or sores on the genitals, such as syphilis or herpes simplex, are at a higher risk for HIV infection. Drug and/or alcohol users also may be at greater risk for infection because these substances often lessen inhibitions and reduce the reluctance to have unsafe, unprotected sex.

Gender and Racial/Ethnic Differences

Annual adult and adolescent rates for AIDS reported in 2003 were far higher for African-Americans (75.2 per one hundred thousand people) and Hispanics (26.8 per one hundred thousand) than for whites (7.2 per one hundred thousand) and Native Americans/Alaska Natives (10.4 per one hundred thousand). The lowest rates were for Asian-Americans and Pacific Islanders (4.8 per one hundred thousand). (See Table 3.10 in Chapter 3.)

More than 8,500 cases of AIDS reported in 2001 were transmitted by IDUs. In 2001 the number had dropped to slightly less than 7,500. By the end of 2003 this reported number had dropped to 7,128. The number of women acquiring AIDS through intravenous drug use in 2000 (2,609), 2001 (2,212), and 2003 (2,262) was less than the number of women who were infected through heterosexual contact (3,981 in 2000, 4,142 in 2001, and 5,234 in 2003). In 2000, 2001, and 2003 about 19, 16, and 15%, respectively, of AIDS cases reported in males was attributable to IDUs, and approximately another 5% (in 2000, 2001, and 2003) were MTM who also injected drugs. (See Table 3.5 in Chapter 3.)

Of the 855 women who became infected with HIV through intravenous drug use during 2000, 53% were African-American, 38% were white, and 7.5% were Hispanic. In 2001 the number of cases of HIV infection that was attributable to IDU had jumped to 1,097. African-Americans accounted for 52%, whites for 33%, and Hispanics for 14% of these cases. Asian-American/Pacific Islander and Native American/Alaska Native women were more likely to be infected through heterosexual contact. In 2003 the number of cases of HIV infection attributable to IDU had increased still more, to 2,262. African-Americans accounted for 17% (1,277), whites for 29% (557), and Hispanics for 18% (385) of cases. Asian-American/Pacific Islander and Hispanic women were more likely to be infected through heterosexual contact. (See Table 3.8 in Chapter 3.)

In men with HIV infection, intravenous drug use was second only to MTM as a risk factor in 2000, 2001, and 2003. Of IDU-exposed men in 2003, 11% were African-American, 19% were Hispanic, 9% were Native American/Alaska

Native, 7% were white, and 5% were Asian-American/ Pacific Islander. (See Table 4.1.)

WOMEN AND AIDS

According to the CDC, the proportion of women among AIDS sufferers has increased steadily, from a reported 7% in 1985 to 23% in June 1999. During 2000, 10,459 American women were diagnosed with AIDS. In 2001 and 2003 the number of cases had risen to 11,082 and 11,561, respectively (*HIV/AIDS Surveillance Report: Cases of HIV Infection and AIDS in the United States, 2003*, vol. 15, Centers for Disease Control and Prevention, 2004).

Fifty-two percent of the 163,396 cumulative 1981– 2003 cases among females were associated either directly or indirectly with intravenous drug use. Of those 85,769 cases, 72% (61,621 cases) occurred among female IDUs, and another 28% (24,148 cases) were among women who reported sexual contact with male IDUs. (See Table 3.5 in Chapter 3.)

Racial/ethnic differences among HIV-infected women and their children are striking. Although African-American and Hispanic women comprise about one-quarter of all U.S. women, they account for 78% of all U.S. women diagnosed with AIDS since 1981 (127,915 cumulative cases of 163,396 reported through 2003). (See Table 3.8 in Chapter 3.)

Women can infect their unborn children with HIV in the course of pregnancy, during delivery, or by breast-feeding after birth. The 48% decrease in the number of women who gave birth to HIV-infected babies during the 1990s was largely attributable to the introduction of the antiretroviral drug zidovudine (ZDV; also known as azi-dothymidine, or AZT). Women of childbearing age can be tested for HIV perinatally (before and during pregnancy), and, if they are positive, have the option of receiving ZDV to prevent passage of the disease to their unborn children.

Along with antiretroviral therapy, which lowers the mother's viral load to undetectable levels, deliveries via elective cesarean section (C-section; the surgical delivery of a baby) rather than vaginal births may also help to reduce mother-to-child transmission. States with HIV case surveillance data are better able to direct resources—targeted public health education programs, health professionals, and prenatal care—aimed at elim-inating prenatal (before birth) transmission of HIV.

HIV/AIDS in Women in Small Towns and Rural Areas

Most HIV/AIDS cases occur among women who live in large metropolitan areas with populations of greater than five hundred thousand. However, the number of HIV/AIDS cases is increasing in rural areas, especially

through heterosexual transmission. A significant number of the more than eighty-one thousand adult and adoles-cent women living with AIDS at the end of 2003 live in southern states. Since a large number lived in states that do not have HIV surveillance, it is likely that there are women who have not been tested. As a result, the num-bers of HIV-infected women may be an underestimate.

Sexually Transmitted Diseases

Prevention, identification, and prompt treatment of STDs are vitally important for the health of young women. Most HIV cases in young women are spread through heterosexual sex (70,200 of the 163,396 total cases in 2003, representing 43%; see Table 3.8 in Chapter 3), and the increase in STDs parallels that of HIV. For instance, the geographic areas with the highest numbers of cases of syphilis and gonorrhea have the highest incidence of cases of HIV among women of childbearing age.

Women with STDs are more likely to become infected with HIV because they have an increased num-ber of HIV target cells (CD4+ T cells) present in their cervical secretions. These cells facilitate the entrance of HIV into the body. Furthermore, women with STDs are more likely to shed HIV in both ulcer-forming and inflammatory genital secretions. They are also more likely to shed HIV in greater amounts than people infected with HIV alone, which contributes to the spread of HIV. By treating an STD, the shedding of HIV on sexual contact is lessened, which in turn reduces the spread of HIV infection.

MALE TO MALE SEXUAL CONTACT

Referred to in the 2003 CDC survey as male to male sexual contact (MTM), this category was previously designated as men having sex with men (MSM). MTM is still the major risk category for HIV infection, although the increase in the number of cases has slowed steadily over the past few years. Epidemiologists (public health researchers who analyze the extent and types of illnesses in a population and the factors that influence their dis-tribution) believe that HIV/AIDS among MTM may have peaked in 1992.

As of December 2000, 44,467 adult and adolescent males whose only stated mode of exposure to HIV was through MTM contact made up 46% of the 97,712 cumu-lative male adult and adolescent HIV infection cases. In 2001 the percentage had fallen slightly, to forty-three. But the actual number of cases attributable to MTM had risen to 52,139 out of a total of 120,868. In 2003, 72,745 reported cases of HIV infection were attributable to MTM, representing 48% of the total of 152,739 cases. (See Table 4.1.)

As in previous years, in 2003 MTM contact is the overwhelming mode of exposure and transmission for non-Hispanic white males with or without intravenous drug use (41,048 cumulative cases, representing 65% of the cumulative total). In 2003 approximately 32% of MTM are comprised of African-American, non-Hispanic males, and 37% are comprised of Hispanic males. Homosexual sex is also the leading mode of HIV exposure for these latter groups. Cumulatively through 2003, 46% of all HIV-infected Hispanic males and 38% of all HIV-infected African-American males had MTM contact, with or without intravenous drug use. (See Table 4.1.)

PRISONERS AND AIDS

According to the Bureau of Justice Statistics' *HIV in Prisons and Jails, 2002* (Laura M. Maruschak, December 2004), the number of HIV-positive prisoners in federal and state prisons grew at about the same rate from 1991 to 1995 as the overall prison population. Between 1995 and 1999 the number of HIV-positive prisoners grew at a slower rate (6%) than the overall prison population (19%). In 1995, however, the rate of HIV/AIDS cases reported among the U.S. prison population (0.51%) was more than six times the rate of the general U.S. public (0.08%). Though this rate of difference has slowly decreased, by 2002 it was still four times the rate of that for the general public (0.14% for the general U.S. population versus 0.48% for state and federal prisoners). (See Table 4.2.) At the end of 2002 the estimated number of confirmed AIDS cases in U.S. prisons stood at 5,643.

Every year since statistics have been gathered, AIDS-related conditions have been the second-leading cause of death for state prison inmates, behind "illness/natural causes." But the proportion of deaths attributable to AIDS has declined markedly since 1995. That year, out of the total number of inmate deaths in state prisons (3,133), 1,569 (50%) were from natural causes other than AIDS and 1,010 (32% of the total) were from AIDS. But by 2002, of the total number of deaths (3,105), 2,405 (77%) were from natural causes other than AIDS while only 215 (7%) were from AIDS. This remarkable decline in AIDS-related deaths is also reflected by the statistics in the rate of deaths per one hundred thousand inmates. In 1995 the death rate in state prisons due to AIDS was one hundred per one hundred thousand inmates; in 2000 the rate had decreased to seventeen per one hundred thousand. (See Table 4.3.) The sharp drop may be the result of effective treatment with protease inhibitors and combination antiretroviral therapies.

A similar trend is also apparent when the inmate death figures from federal prisons in 2001 and 2002 are examined. Of the total number of inmate deaths in federal prisons in 2001 (303), 247 (82%) were from natural causes other than AIDS, and twenty-two (7%) were from AIDS. By the following year, 289 out of a total of 335

TABLE 4.2

Percentage of general and prison populations with confirmed AIDS, 1995–2002

	Percent of population with confirmed AIDS	
Year	U.S. general population	State and federal prisoners
1995	0.08%	0.51%
1996	0.09	0.54
1997	0.10	0.55
1998	0.11	0.53
1999	0.12	0.60
2000	0.13	0.53
2001	0.14	0.52
2002	0.14	0.48

Note: The percent of the general population with confirmed AIDS in each year may be overestimated due to delays in death reports.

SOURCE: Laura M. Maruschak, "Percentage of Population with Confirmed AIDS," in *HIV in Prisons and Jails, 2002*, Bureau of Justice Statistics, December 2004, http://www.ojp.usdoj.gov/bjs/pub/pdf/hivpj02.pdf (accessed July 18, 2005)

TABLE 4.3

Inmate deaths in state prisons, by cause, 1995 and 2002

	Deaths of state inmates			
	Number*		Rate per 100,000 inmates	
Cause of death	2002	1995	2002	1995
Total	**3,105**	**3,133**	**246**	**311**
Natural causes other than AIDS	2,405	1,569	190	156
AIDS	215	1,010	17	100
Suicide	166	160	13	16
Accident	41	48	3	5
Execution	70	56	6	6
By another person	53	86	4	9
Other/unspecified	155	204	12	20

*Detail may not add to total due to rounding.

SOURCE: Laura M. Maruschak, "Table 4. Inmate Deaths in State Prisons, by Cause, 1995 and 2002," in *HIV in Prisons and Jails, 2002*, Bureau of Justice Statistics, December 2004, http://www.ojp.usdoj.gov/bjs/pub/pdf/hivpj02.pdf (accessed July 18, 2005)

deaths (86%) were from natural causes other than AIDS, while seventeen (5%) were from AIDS. (See Table 4.4.) The decline is more modest than the data for state prisons because the data for federal prisons was compiled over two years instead of seven.

Geographic Differences

At the conclusion of 2002, 23,864 U.S. inmates were confirmed as being infected with HIV, according to the Bureau of Justice Statistics (BJS). This represents 1.9% of the custody population at that time—a decrease from the 2.2% of inmates known to be HIV-infected in 1998. This modest decrease has not been geographically uniform, however. At year end 2002, New York State held a fifth of all inmates (5,000, or 21%) known to be

TABLE 4.4

Inmate deaths in federal prisons, by cause, 2001–02

| | Deaths of federal inmates | | | |
| | Number | | Rate per 100,000 inmates | |
Cause of death	2002	2001	2002	2001
Total	335	303	207	198
Natural causes other than AIDS	289	247	179	162
AIDS	17	22	11	14
Suicide	17	18	11	12
Accident	5	6	3	4
Execution	0	2	0	1
By another person	3	8	2	5
Other/unspecified	4	0	2	0

*Detail may not add to total due to rounding.

SOURCE: Laura M. Maruschak, "Table 5. Inmate Deaths in Federal Prisons, by Cause, 2001 and 2002," in *HIV in Prisons and Jails, 2002*, Bureau of Justice Statistics, December 2004, http://www.ojp.usdoj.gov/bjs/pub/pdf/hivpj02.pdf (accessed July 18, 2005)

TABLE 4.5

Number of HIV-infected prison inmates, 1998–2002

Jurisdiction	Number	Percent of custody population
New York	5,000	7.5%
Florida	2,848	3.8
Texas	2,528	1.9
Federal system	1,547	1.1
California	1,181	0.7
Georgia	1,123	2.4

SOURCE: Laura M. Maruschak, "Highlights. Number of HIV-Infected Inmates Steadily Decreasing since 1999," in *HIV in Prisons and Jails, 2002*, Bureau of Justice Statistics, December 2004, http://www.ojp.usdoj.gov/bjs/pub/pdf/hivpj02.pdf (accessed July 18, 2005)

TABLE 4.6

Profile of inmates who died in state prisons, 2001–02

| Characteristic | Number of AIDS-related deaths | | AIDS-related deaths per 100,000 inmates | |
	2002	2001	2002	2001
State total	283	311	22	25
Reported in DICRA	245	270	20	23
Gender				
Male	236	256	21	23
Female	9	14	11	18
Age				
24 or younger	0	4	0	2
25–34	28	45	6	10
35–44	119	130	34	37
45 or older	98	91	64	61
Race/Hispanic origin				
White	50	49	12	11
Black	163	181	30	33
Hispanic	30	40	15	24

SOURCE: Laura M. Maruschak, "Table 7. Profile of Inmates Who Died in State Prisons, 2001 and 2002," in *HIV in Prisons and Jails, 2002*, Bureau of Justice Statistics, December 2004, http://www.ojp.usdoj.gov/bjs/pub/pdf/hivpj02.pdf (accessed July 18, 2005)

HIV-positive. In contrast, California held 5% (1,181) of all HIV-positive inmates. (See Table 4.5.)

Gender, Racial, and Age Differences

At the end of 2002 an estimated 5,643 U.S. inmates had confirmed cases of AIDS, according to the BJS. This was a decrease from the estimated 6,809 cases confirmed in 1999.

This decrease was not uniform for males and females. Of the total U.S. prison population in 2002, 3% of female inmates were known to be HIV-positive, in contrast to 1.9% of male inmates. The increased infection rate for females was not mirrored in the number of AIDS-related deaths, however. In state prisons in both 2001 and 2002, the number of male deaths (256 and 236, respectively) was far greater than the number of female AIDS-related deaths (fourteen and nine, respectively). (See Table 4.6.)

BJS statistics from state prisons also reveal age and racial differences. The number of deaths in state prisons in 2001 and 2002 was greatest for thirty-five to forty-four-year-olds (130 and 119, respectively), followed by the forty-five and older age group (ninety-one and ninety-eight, respectively). Fewer deaths were evident in the twenty-five to thirty-four age category (forty-five and twenty-eight, respectively). (See Table 4.6.)

Statistics obtained from local jails reveal similar trends. In 2000, 2001, and 2002 male deaths (fifty-three, fifty-one, and thirty-eight, respectively) greatly exceeded the number of female deaths in the same years (five, four, and four, respectively). The thirty-five to forty-four age group experienced more deaths than the other age groups, and the number of deaths of African-Americans was four to eight times more than that of whites and Hispanics. (See Table 4.7.)

Statistics from 2002 indicate that the current reason for incarceration is not associated with a prisoner's HIV-positive status. But a history of prior drug use is associated with whether or not a prisoner is HIV-positive. Only 0.4% of the 51,248 prisoners who were drug-free were HIV-positive, in contrast to 3.2% of the 66,606 prisoners who had used a needle to inject drugs and 7.5% of prisoners who shared a needle in drug injection. (See Table 4.8.)

Testing Policies in U.S. Prisons

Guidelines for the testing of inmates for HIV exist in all fifty states, the District of Columbia, and the regulations of the Federal Bureau of Prisons. But the timing of

TABLE 4.7

Profile of inmates who died in local jails, 2000–02

	Number of AIDS-related deaths			AIDS-related deaths per 100,000 inmates		
Characteristic	2002	2001	2000	2002	2001	2000
All inmates	42	55	58	6	9	9
Gender						
Male	38	51	53	6	9	10
Female	4	4	5	5	5	7
Age						
24 or younger	1	2	0	1	1	0
25–34	11	13	16	0	5	7
35–44	21	26	22	12	17	14
45 or older	9	14	20	11	28	40
Race/Hispanic origin						
White	5	5	10	2	2	4
Black	31	39	43	12	15	17
Hispanic	5	10	5	5	11	5

SOURCE: Laura M. Maruschak, "Table 11. Profile of Inmates Who Died in Local Jails, 2000–2002," in *HIV in Prisons and Jails, 2002*, Bureau of Justice Statistics, December 2004, http://www.ojp.usdoj.gov/bjs/pub/pdf/hivpj02.pdf (accessed July 18, 2005)

TABLE 4.8

Results of HIV tests among jail inmates, by offense and prior drug use, 2002

	Tested inmates who reported results	
Characteristic	Number	Percent HIV positive
Current offense		
Violent	90,751	0.7%
Property	95,599	1.8
Drug	96,003	1.6
Public-order	87,374	1.1
Prior drug use		
Never used	51,248	0.4%
Ever used	322,617	1.5
Used month before offense	162,027	1.5
Used needle to inject drugs	66,606	3.2
Share a needle	22,288	7.5

SOURCE: Laura M. Maruschak, "Table 10. Results of Tests for the Human Immunodeficiency Virus among Jail Inmates, by Offense and Prior Drug Use, 2002," in *HIV in Prisons and Jails, 2002*, Bureau of Justice Statistics, December 2004, http://www.ojp.usdoj.gov/bjs/pub/pdf/hivpj02.pdf (accessed July 18, 2005)

testing varies. As of 2003 nineteen of the fifty-two jurisdictions tested prisoners entering the prison system, and three states plus federal prisons tested prisoners on their release. Forty-five jurisdictions and federal prisons tested prisoners if inmates request a test; forty-five jurisdictions plus federal prisons tested inmates if they display HIV-related symptoms. Forty states and all federal facilities tested prisoners after they have been involved in incidents such as fights, and fifteen states tested inmates who have been classified as "high risk."

The testing guidelines adhere to the policy on management of infectious diseases that is detailed in a 2005 Program Statement (Number P6190.03) of the Department of Justice's Federal Bureau of Prisons. Testing can be performed on a voluntary basis, when requested by an inmate. But if there is concern over the possibility of infection or exposure to HIV, testing is mandatory, and can override inmate objections. All inmates who are tested receive pre- and post-test counseling, even if they test negative. This helps to increase awareness of HIV and AIDS and deter the spread of the infection through inmate populations.

HIV testing of prisoners is controversial in many states because of patient confidentiality laws that require medical test results to be kept secret. In Washington State, concern for prison guards' health prompted the passage of legislation almost a decade ago that allows corrections workers who have been exposed to a prisoner's bodily fluids to find out if that prisoner tested positive for STDs, including HIV.

Drug and Needle Use among Prisoners

Public education campaigns about the "safer" use of drugs and syringes appear to be reducing HIV infection in the general public. In contrast, these measures seem to be having no effect in prisons. Many incarcerated IDUs continue to inject while in prison, often sharing needles because injection equipment is in short supply. Indeed, more than 70% of incarcerated IDUs reported borrowing syringes while in prison. The consequences of this behavior are evident in the high rate of HIV infection among prisoners who shared a needle for drug injection prior to incarceration (7.5%, representing 1,672 of 22,288 HIV-positive inmates, according to BJS statistics from 2002). (See Table 4.8.)

This is a dilemma for prisons, where syringes and needles are prohibited, as are illegal drugs, and chemicals for disinfecting the illicit needles are not readily available to prisoners. While state and federal prison officials in the United States want to stop the spread of HIV among inmates, most cannot keep pace with or stem the flow of illegal drugs into prisons. To minimize the spread of HIV in prisons, countries such as Switzerland and the United Kingdom provide prisoners with disinfectant or clean needles. U.S. officials believe that these actions endorse illegal drug use. Instead, they focus on providing treatment and rehabilitation programs for drug-addicted prisoners.

HEMOPHILIACS

Hemophilia is a group of genetic disorders in which defects in a number of genes located on the X chromosome disrupt the proper clotting of blood. The most common type of hemophilia—hemophilia A—is a deficiency of a clotting substance designated Factor VIII. Varying severities of hemophilia can occur, depending on the level of Factor VIII present in the patient's plasma. Treatment of hemophilia involves close attention to injury prevention and periodic intravenous administration of Factor VIII concentrates, commonly known as clotting factors.

Because screening for HIV antibodies was not available until 1985, many hemophiliacs were exposed to HIV-contaminated blood and clotting factors prior to widespread use of screening procedures. National distribution of clotting factor concentrates prior to 1985 led to a high prevalence of HIV infections among hemophiliacs. The prevalence of HIV infection differs by the type and severity of the coagulation (clotting) disorder.

According to the CDC, as of December 2003, 5,448 adult, adolescent, and pediatric hemophiliacs had been diagnosed with AIDS in the United States, representing 1% of the total AIDS population. While statistics are unavailable, many health officials believe that 70 to 90% of the approximately seventeen thousand Americans with hemophilia A are HIV-positive. The eight thousand or so Americans with the less clinically severe hemophilia B most likely have a lower prevalence rate because they required fewer treatments with the clotting factor and, therefore, were less exposed to HIV-contaminated products. Hemophilia A rates may be overrepresented, according to the CDC, since the studies were performed at hemophilia treatment centers where the more severe hemophilia A cases are likely to be found.

Prior to the 1980s, most hemophiliacs died from intracranial hemorrhage (bleeding within the brain). But by 1995 one-third of all deaths were related to HIV infection while one-fourth were related to hemorrhage. Hemophiliacs often report that virtually all their fellow hemophiliacs are infected with the virus. Many sexual partners of hemophiliacs have also contracted the virus

from sexual intercourse. In the case of females, the virus can subsequently be passed to their offspring.

A Slow Reaction

Concentrated clotting factor, which is derived from human blood obtained from as many as two thousand donors, became available in the mid-1970s. Its success at stopping bleeding was so dramatic that hemophilia changed from a disease that produced intense pain, disability, and the possibility of premature death to one that allowed sufferers to lead nearly normal lives. Hemophiliacs could infuse clotting factors into their own veins if they felt bleeding was about to start. Patients were advised by their physicians to "infuse early and often."

Disastrously, during the late 1970s and early 1980s some clotting factor concentrates were infected with HIV. Even after the first cases of HIV/AIDS appeared in people with hemophilia and the CDC, along with the Hemophiliac Foundation, identified this new disease as being blood-borne, physicians did not advise their patients to alter their clotting factor treatments. Hemophiliacs were encouraged to continue using their clotting factor because Hemophilia Foundation officials were not sure there would be a major epidemic.

Anecdotal comments from hemophiliacs indicate that when many of them became infected, primary care doctors were slow to respond and supplied very little information. There was no warning to practice "safe sex" to prevent the spread of HIV. Some hemophiliacs reported receiving more information from gay men's organizations than from their own hematologists (physicians who specialize in diseases and disorders of the blood).

ANGER AND COMPENSATION. Many hemophiliacs feel they are entitled to compensation or, at the very least, assistance in paying their overwhelming medical expenses. They maintain that the companies that produced the clotting factors were slow to warn the public about HIV and slow to use heat treatment to eliminate the live virus from the clotting factors (although this procedure has not gained widespread acceptance among scientists as an adequate method to inactivate HIV).

Hemophilia foundations in some countries have convinced governments or insurance companies to compensate HIV-infected hemophiliacs. Japan agreed to pay $1,500 a month to affected patients; Canada offered each patient a lump sum of $120,000 (although legal arguments have delayed this compensation); Denmark will pay $42,500; and Britain $30,000 a person. France dispenses funds from its $5.5 billion pool to hemophiliacs who were infected with HIV/AIDS because of tainted blood products.

The U.S. government has no plans to compensate people with HIV/AIDS and hemophilia, and in 1995 the U.S. Supreme Court refused to hear a class action suit brought by hemophiliacs against a pharmaceutical company and other blood product manufacturers (*Barton v. American Red Cross*, 826 F. Supp. 412 and 826 F. Supp. 407. Append 43 F. 3rd 678. Certiori denied 116 S. Ct. 84). Nonetheless, some companies have reached out-of-court settlements with affected people. In May 1996 four manufacturers of blood clotting products offered $640 million to an estimated six thousand people.

CHAPTER 5

CHILDREN, ADOLESCENTS, AND HIV/AIDS

HIV/AIDS IN CHILDREN—DIFFERENT FROM HIV/AIDS IN ADULTS

HIV causes AIDS in both adults and children. The virus attacks and damages the immune and central nervous systems of all infected people. But the development and course of the disease in children differs considerably from its progression in adults.

Before the use of highly active antiretroviral therapy (HAART) and early intervention strategies, there were two patterns of HIV progression among children. The first pattern, which is called severe immunodeficiency, is apparent as recurring serious infections or encephalopathy (a disease of the brain). Severe immunodeficiency develops in 15 to 20% of infected infants during their first year of life. The second pattern of HIV progression, which occurs in the other 80 to 85% of infected children, is more gradual and is similar to the development seen in adults.

HIV nucleic acid detection tests can detect the presence of HIV in nearly all infants ages one month or older. Prior to the development of these tests, detecting HIV infection, especially in babies, was difficult. This is because the earlier tests involved the detection of antibodies formed by the infant in response to HIV. But infants have often not developed the full capacity to produce antibodies at the time of testing. Furthermore, HIV-infected mothers may transmit antibodies alone, without the virus, to their babies. In the latter instance, infants with positive results from antibody tests at birth may later test negative, indicating that the mother transmitted the HIV antibodies to the baby, but not the virus itself.

In adults, symptoms of fully developed AIDS include the presence of opportunistic infections (OIs) that may or may not be accompanied by rare forms of several types of cancers. The OIs or the cancers can ultimately prove to be the cause of death. The most common diseases associated with AIDS in adults are *Pneumocystis carinii* pneumonia (PCP) and Kaposi's sarcoma. The latter is a normally rare skin carcinoma that is capable of spreading to internal organs. Many adult AIDS patients have one or both of these conditions. Other disorders found in adult AIDS patients are lymphomas (lymph gland cancers), prolonged diarrhea causing severe dehydration, weight loss, and central nervous system infections that can lead to dementia.

Among infants and children, the disease is characterized by wasting syndrome, the failure to thrive, and unusually severe bacterial infections. With the exception of PCP, children with symptomatic HIV infection rarely develop the same OIs that adults contract. Though adults and children with HIV may both suffer from chronic or recurrent diarrhea, its dehydrating effect may be particularly debilitating and life-threatening to children. Instead of other symptoms common to adults, children are plagued with recurrent bacterial infections and persistent or recurrent oral thrush (an infection of the mouth or throat caused by the fungus *Candida albicans*). Children may also suffer from enlarged lymph nodes, chronic pneumonia, developmental delays, and neurological abnormalities. Tragically, the immune system of HIV-infected children is destroyed even as it matures.

Whether HIV-positive or not, babies born to HIV-infected mothers appear to be predisposed to a variety of heart problems. In a study published in the journal *The Lancet* in June 2002, Steven Lipshultz et al. at Harvard Medical School examined more than five hundred infants born to HIV-positive women. They discovered that the babies suffered from abnormalities, such as defects in the heart wall and valve and reduced pumping action. These defects occur in less than 1% of healthy children whose mothers are not infected with HIV. Lipshultz and his colleagues recognize that HIV alone did not necessarily cause these anomalies. A mother's alcohol, drug, or nutrition problems, they observe, can also interfere with fetal heart development.

A CASE DEFINITION FOR CHILDREN

Because there was limited data during the first few years of HIV's acknowledged presence in the United States, the Centers for Disease Control and Prevention (CDC) definition of AIDS did not differentiate between adults and children until 1987, when the classification system was revised. The CDC updated the pediatric definition in 1994 and again in 1999 as more information about HIV and AIDS became available. The revisions, which remain current in 2005, are intended to:

- Reflect the stage of disease for an HIV-infected child

- Balance simplicity and medical accuracy in the classification process

- Establish mutually exclusive classification categories

As summarized in Table 5.1, HIV-infected children are classified clinically using a series of categories that range from the absence of symptoms (N1) to a severe manifestation of the symptoms (C3). The symptoms used in these classifications relate to the evidence and degrees of suppression of the immune system. The diagnosis and case definitions of HIV infection in children are based on a number of test results and HIV infection definition criteria in mutually exclusive categories according to three parameters: infection status, clinical status, and immunologic status. (See Table 5.2, and Table 2.3 in Chapter 2.)

As of December 1999 the diagnostic criteria for HIV infection in children eighteen months or younger

TABLE 5.1

Pediatric HIV classification[a]

Immunologic categories	Clinical categories			
	N: No signs/ symptoms	A: Mild signs/ symptoms	B:[b] Moderate signs/ symptoms	C:[b] Severe signs/ symptoms
1: No evidence of suppression	N1	A1	B1	C1
2: Evidence of moderate suppression	N2	A2	B2	C2
3: Severe suppression	N3	A3	B3	C3

[a]Children whose HIV infection status is not confirmed are classified by using the above grid with a letter E (for perinatally exposed) placed before the appropriate classification code (e.g., EN 2)
[b]Both Category C and lymphoid interstitial pneumonitis in Category B are reportable to state and local health departments as acquired immunodeficiency syndrome.

SOURCE: "Table 1. Pediatric Human Immunodeficiency Virus (HIV) Classification," in "1994 Revised Classification System for HIV Infection in Children Less Than 13 Years of Age; Official Authorized Addenda: Human Immunodeficiency Virus Infection Codes and Official Guidelines for Coding and Reporting ICD-9-CM," in *Morbidity and Mortality Weekly Report: Recommendations and Reports*, vol. 43, no. RR-12, September 30, 1994

TABLE 5.2

Diagnosis of HIV infection in children*

Diagnosis: HIV-infected

a) A child <18 months of age who is known to be HIV seropositive or born to an HIV-infected mother **and**:

- has positive results on two separate determinations (excluding cord blood) from one or more of the following HIV detection tests:
— HIV culture,
— HIV polymerase chain reaction,
— HIV antigen (p24)

or

- meets criteria for acquired immunodeficiency syndrome (AIDS) diagnosis based on the 1987 AIDS surveillance case definition (10)

b) A child >18 months of age born to an HIV-infected mother or any child infected by blood, blood products, or other known modes of transmission (e.g., sexual contact) who: —

- is HIV-antibody positive by repeatedly reactive enzyme immunoassay (EIA) and confirmatory test (e.g., Western blot or immunoflurescence assy [IFA]);

or

- meets any of the criteria in a) above.

Diagnosis: Perinatally exposed (prefix E)

A child who does not meet the criteria above who:

- is HIV seropositive by EIA and confirmatory test (e.g., Western blot or IFA) and is <18 months of age at the time of test:

or

- has unknown antibody status, but was born to a mother known to be infected with HIV.

Diagnosis: Seroreverter (SR)

A child who is born to an HIV-infected mother and who:

- has been documented as HIV-antibody negative (i.e., two or more negative EIA tests performed at 6–18 months of age or one negative EIA test after 18 months of age);

and

- has had no other laboratory evidence of infection (has not had two positive viral detection tests, if performed);

and

- has not had an AIDS-defining condition.

*This definition of HIV infection replaces the definition published in the 1987 AIDS surveillance case definition (10).

SOURCE: "Box 1. Diagnosis of Human Immunodeficiency Virus (HIV) Infection in Children," in "1994 Revised Classification System for HIV Infection in Children Less Than 13 Years of Age; Official Authorized Addenda: Human Immunodeficiency Virus Infection Codes and Official Guidelines for Coding and Reporting ICD-9-CM," in *Morbidity and Mortality Weekly Report: Recommendations and Reports*, vol. 43, no. RR-12, September 30, 1994

requires positive results from HIV nucleic acid testing, HIV p24 antigen testing for children one month or older, or the actual isolation of HIV using viral culture-based methods. (See Table 2.3 in Chapter 2.) Prior to the availability of HIV nucleic acid detection tests, which do not rely on the detection of antibodies, cases of HIV infection in infants were difficult to diagnose accurately. This is because using tests to identify anti-HIV antibodies, which move through the placenta into the fetus, can complicate diagnosis of HIV infection in children born to infected mothers. Almost all children born to HIV-infected mothers test positive for the HIV antibody at their birth, even though only 15 to 30% are actually infected. In uninfected babies the HIV antibody usually becomes undetectable by nine months, although it may remain detectable for up to eighteen months.

There are three categories of HIV-infected children: those younger than eighteen months who are perinatally exposed (acquired the virus from their mother); children older than eighteen months with perinatal infection; and infants and children of all ages who acquired the virus through other types of exposure.

Children Younger Than Eighteen Months

The screening and confirmatory blood tests that accurately diagnose HIV in adults are not reliable for detecting HIV in children younger than eighteen months old because of the presence of passively acquired maternal antibodies. Early recognition of HIV infection in infants younger than eighteen months is accomplished using polymerase chain reaction (PCR), a test that amplifies amounts of viral genetic material to detectable levels, by the direct isolation of the HIV virus using viral culture techniques, or by the detection of the p24 viral antigen. These tests can identify 30 to 50% of infected babies at birth and almost 100% by three to six months of age. Those who are HIV-antibody positive and asymptomatic (without symptoms) without immune abnormalities have an HIV infection status that cannot be determined unless a virus culture or other antigen-detection test is positive. As with any diagnostic test, accuracy of detection is not absolute. The test does not detect 100% of people who are HIV-positive. Low levels of virus may escape detection. This possibility of a "false negative" result means that a negative culture does not necessarily rule out an infection. A small percentage of people who are infected with HIV can produce a negative result on testing.

Infants and children who are known to have been perinatally exposed (in other words, their mother is known to be HIV-positive) but who lack one of the diagnostic criteria for HIV infection should be observed further for HIV-related illnesses and tested at regular intervals. The U.S. Public Health Service recommends that all infants of HIV-infected mothers be given the drug zidovudine (ZDV) for six weeks and that HIV-infected mothers be warned about the risks of transmission through breastfeeding. Infants with negative HIV tests at birth should be retested periodically during the first eighteen months of life. Studies suggest that ZDV therapy does not influence the accuracy of virus detection tests and consequently does not delay diagnosis of HIV infection.

Older Children

HIV infection in older children is defined by one or more of the following:

- Identification of the virus in the blood or tissues

- The presence of HIV antibodies (positive screening plus confirmatory test), regardless of the presence of immunologic abnormalities or symptoms

- Confirmation that symptoms meet the previously published CDC case definition for HIV infection

PERINATAL INFECTION

More than 90% of the cumulative totals of children younger than thirteen who have been reported to have HIV infection through 2003 were infected perinatally. A number of factors are associated with an increased risk of an HIV-positive mother passing the infection to her fetus. They include low CD4+ T cell count, high viral load (the concentration of virus in the blood), advanced HIV progression, presence of a particular HIV protein (p24) in serum, and placental membrane inflammation. Intrapartum (at the time of birth) events resulting in increased exposure of the fetus to maternal blood, breastfeeding, low vitamin A levels, premature rupture of membranes, prenatal use of illicit drugs, and premature delivery also increase the risk of mother-to-fetus transmission. The risk of perinatal transmission also increases when the mother does not know she is infected until late in the course of the illness.

Despite these potential routes of transmission, the number of HIV-infected infants has been declining, probably as a result of the more widespread use of HAART to prevent pregnant women from passing HIV infection to their offspring. Planned cesarean section delivery (C-section), the presence of neutralizing antibodies in the mother, and timely antiviral drug therapy (such as with ZDV) further reduce the chances of mother-to-infant HIV transmission.

There is evidence that planned C-section, the procedure where a fetus is delivered by surgical removal from the womb, together with the administration of ZDV, may prevent some cases of mother-to-baby HIV infection. C-section delivery does not expose the fetus to potentially HIV-contaminated vaginal tissue.

ZDV

Even without a C-section, drug therapy can be beneficial. In the United States and Western Europe the number of babies born with HIV infection has been reduced 50% by giving infected pregnant women and their newborns ZDV. Before widespread use of ZDV, about five hundred American babies per year, nearly all of them either African-American or Hispanic, were infected with HIV from their mothers. By 2003 there were only 147 reported cases of mother-to-child transmission in the United States. Worldwide, nine thousand babies are born annually who are infected with HIV. Infection usually occurs during the last stages of pregnancy, most often during labor and delivery. There is evidence in the scientific literature that planned cesarean delivery, together with the administration of ZDV, may prevent more cases of mother-to-baby HIV infection.

TREATMENTS FOR CHILDREN

Prescribing drug therapy for children is often more difficult than prescribing for adults because children respond to drugs differently at different ages and because oral medication must have an acceptable taste to children so that they will take it as prescribed.

As of January 2004 twelve antiretroviral drugs had been approved for pediatric HIV patients by the U.S. Food and Drug Administration (FDA). Of these, four drugs called protease inhibitors (PIs; used alone or in combination with other drugs to combat viral infection) were available to children two to thirteen years old. They are nelfinavir, ritonavir, amprenavir, and lopinavir/ritonavir. PI compounds act by preventing the reproduction of HIV that is already in the host cells.

Another group of drugs approved for pediatric use are known as nucleoside analogs (NAs). NAs, which are structurally similar to a nucleoside constituent of DNA, limit HIV replication by incorporating themselves into a strand of DNA, which causes the chain to end. The NAs presently approved for pediatric use (the initial FDA approval is denoted in parentheses; this date in some cases pre-dates the approval for pediatric use) are:

- Zidovudine (ZDV), sold under the brand name Retrovir (1987)

- Didanosine (ddI), sold under the brand name Videx (1989)

- Lamivudine (3TC), sold under the brand name Epivir (1995)

- Stavudine (d4T), sold under the brand name Zerit (1994)

- Abacavir Succinate, sold under the brand name Ziagen (1998)

Another group of antiretroviral drugs are known as nonnucleoside reverse transcriptase inhibitors (NNRTIs). NNRTIs slow down the functioning of the enzyme that allows the virus to become a part of the infected cell's nucleus. Two NNRTIs are presently approved for pediatric use:

- Nevirapine, sold under the brand name Viramune (1996)

- Efavirenz, sold under the brand name Sustiva; in Europe efavirenz is sold under the brand name Stocrin (1998)

In 2003 the drug Enfuvirtide was approved for use by children over the age of six. This drug is the first of the fusion inhibitor class of antiretroviral drugs. It acts by inhibiting the fusion of HIV to the host cell membrane.

In March 1996 the Antiviral Drugs Advisory Committee of the FDA approved the use of the compound didanosine (ddI; brand name Videx) for pediatric use. The drug was developed and is marketed by Bristol-Myers Squibb Pharmaceuticals. The approval was based on the results of two separate U.S. AIDS Clinical Trials Group pediatric studies (one of which was the largest controlled pediatric trial to date) and an Australian study, all of which found that Videx delayed the progression of AIDS and was superior to ZDV alone. ZDV, which is given to children and adults, had been the only drug widely recognized to help delay the progress of HIV infection and to reduce the risk of perinatal infection.

The study results generated high expectations for the performance of Videx in both children and adults. Indeed, the Videx and combination therapies were so much more effective than ZDV alone that the AIDS Clinical Trial Group prematurely discontinued the ZDV-only therapy portion of the study. As promising as these early reports seemed, the effectiveness of Videx alone or in combination with ZDV was short lived because HIV susceptibility to the drugs decreased over time. Thus, while Videx is still used, it has not been a major breakthrough in HIV infections as was hoped.

In 1999 a study conducted jointly between the United States and Uganda demonstrated that the perinatal transmission of HIV from mother to child could be reduced by the drug nevirapine. The drug is given to the mother in labor and to the child within three days of birth. Initial study results showed the drug to be safe for both mother and child and relatively inexpensive ($4 per mother/child dose). In 2000 the Elizabeth Glaser Pediatric AIDS Foundation, a nonprofit organization dedicated to promoting and funding worldwide pediatric AIDS research, secured funds to implement this treatment in developing countries that lack health care resources and infrastructure.

By 2003 the administration of nevirapine to hundreds of thousands of pregnant women in Africa demonstrated the therapeutic potential of the drug in slowing the progression of pediatric AIDS. The World Health Organization (WHO), governments throughout sub-Saharan Africa, and the U.S. National Institutes of Health have all recommended that nevirapine use be continued to prevent HIV transmission from mothers to infants.

HOW MANY CHILDREN ARE INFECTED?

Of the 35,301 cases of HIV infection reported in the United States in 2003, 459 were diagnosed in children younger than thirteen. (See Table 5.3.) The CDC estimates that between six thousand and seven thousand infants every year are born to HIV-infected women in the United

TABLE 5.3

Reported cases of HIV infection, by age category, transmission category, and sex, cumulative through 2003

Transmission category	Males 2003 No.	%	Males Cumulative through 2003* No.	%	Females 2003 No.	%	Females Cumulative through 2003* No.	%	Total 2003 No.	%	Total Cumulative through 2003* No.	%
Adult or adolescent												
Male-to-male sexual contact	10,466	46	72,745	48	—	—	—	—	10,466	32	72,745	34
Injection drug use	2,551	11	19,652	13	1,355	14	11,480	18	3,906	12	31,133	14
Male-to-male sexual contact and injection drug use	732	3	8,623	6	—	—	—	—	732	2	8,623	4
Hemophilia/coagulation disorder	48	0	520	0	12	0	64	0	60	0	584	0
Heterosexual contact	2,009	9	12,669	8	4,036	40	28,483	45	6,045	18	41,152	19
Sex with injection drug user	307	1	2,272	1	628	6	5,901	9	935	3	8,173	4
Sex with bisexual male					193	2	1,757	3	193	1	1,757	1
Sex with person with hemophilia	6	0	25	0	12	0	174	0	18	0	199	0
Sex with HIV-infected transfusion recipient	15	0	116	0	14	0	175	0	29	0	291	0
Sex with HIV-infected person, risk factor not specified	1,681	7	10,256	7	3,189	32	20,476	32	4,870	15	30,732	14
Receipt of blood transfusion, blood components, or tissue	26	0	477	0	61	1	539	1	87	0	1,016	0
Other/risk factor not reported or identified	7,003	31	38,053	25	4,543	45	23,174	36	11,546	35	61,233	28
Subtotal	22,835	100	152,739	100	10,007	100	63,740	100	32,842	100	216,486	100
Child (<13 years at diagnosis)												
Hemophilia/coagulation disorder	5	2	107	5	0	0	1	0	5	1	108	2
Mother with the following risk factor for, or documented, HIV infection:	170	74	1,898	83	152	66	2,000	87	322	70	3,898	85
Injection drug use	19	8	516	23	23	10	518	23	42	9	1,034	23
Sex with injection drug user	14	6	197	9	8	3	196	9	22	5	393	9
Sex with bisexual male	3	1	26	1	2	1	18	1	5	1	44	1
Sex with person with hemophilia	0	0	2	0	0	0	7	0	0	0	9	0
Sex with HIV-infected transfusion recipient	0	0	6	0	0	0	5	0	0	0	11	0
Sex with HIV-infected person, risk factor not specified	58	25	422	19	34	15	483	21	92	20	905	20
Receipt of blood transfusion, blood components, or tissue	1	0	17	1	1	0	16	1	2	0	33	1
Has HIV infection, risk factor not specified	75	33	712	31	84	37	757	33	159	35	1,469	32
Receipt of blood transfusion, blood components, or tissue	2	1	24	1	2	1	27	1	4	1	51	1
Other/risk factor not reported or identified	53	23	252	11	75	33	270	12	128	28	522	11
Subtotal	230	100	2,281	100	229	100	2,298	100	459	100	4,579	100
Total	**23,065**	**100**	**155,020**	**100**	**10,236**	**100**	**66,038**	**100**	**33,301**	**100**	**221,065**	**100**

Note: Includes only persons with HIV infection that has not progressed to AIDS.

* Includes persons with a diagnosis of HIV infection (not AIDS), reported from the beginning of the epidemic through December 2003. Cumulative total includes 7 persons of unknown sex.

SOURCE: "Table 18. Reported Cases of HIV Infection (Not AIDS), by Age Category, Transmission Category, and Sex, Cumulative through 2003—United States," in *HIV/AIDS Surveillance Report: Cases of HIV Infection and AIDS in the United States, 2003*, vol. 15, Centers for Disease Control and Prevention, 2004, http://www.cdc.gov/hiv/stats/2003SurveillanceReport.pdf (accessed July 18, 2005)

States. Of the ninety pediatric HIV cases reported in 2003, fifteen of which were diagnosed with AIDS, sixty-two cases (representing 69% of the total) were in African-American children. (See Table 3.11 in Chapter 3.)

Age at Diagnosis

In 1999 the CDC reported that more than 90% of children with AIDS acquired the disease perinatally and were diagnosed before they were five years old. Four percent were exposed through transfusions, 3% had hemophilia/coagulation disorders, and 2% had no identified or reported risk factors.

Geographic Distribution

In 2003 the CDC-reported geographic distribution of the rate of pediatric and adult/adolescent AIDS cases per one hundred thousand population was very similar, with a higher prevalence in New York (10.5 for pediatric AIDS and 417.9 for adult/adolescent AIDS), Florida (12.8 and 301.9), Pennsylvania (6.1 and 145.4), and New Jersey (19.0 and 214.2). In other states the prevalence of both pediatric and adult/adolescent AIDS was lower, such as in Alaska (1.5 and 52.3), Maine (1.6 and 46.2), Montana (0 and 22.8), North Dakota (1.0 and 10.5), South Dakota (0.7 and 16.5), and Nebraska (1.3 and 41.6).

Worldwide, HIV infection is particularly prevalent in developing countries that lack health care infrastructure, according to the Elizabeth Glaser Pediatric AIDS Foundation. The foundation claims that such countries may have HIV infection rates among pregnant women as high as 25 to 40%. Because these women do not have access to prenatal medical care, prevention programs, and other health care, their babies have a 15 to 30% chance of becoming infected.

SOME CHILDREN BEAT THE VIRUS

Although very rare, infants born to HIV-positive mothers, and who themselves are initially infected with the virus, can subsequently become HIV-negative, develop immunological tolerance to the infection, or segregate the virus in lymphatic (located in the lymph nodes) tissue, where it remains dormant.

The molecular underpinnings of this resistance mechanism, if that is indeed what it proves to be, are as yet unknown. Scientists still do not know the mechanism that triggers this apparent HIV-positive to HIV-negative reversal. Interest in people who convert from HIV positive is high because by identifying the mechanism by which HIV-positive infants clear the virus may help to develop more effective treatments, including immunization against HIV infection.

Gene Mutation in Some Babies May Help

A gene mutation that slows the progress of HIV in adults was shown in the late 1990s to help HIV-infected newborns avoid serious AIDS-associated illnesses longer than those who do not have the mutation. The gene, called CC chemokine receptor 5 (CCR5), is present in 10 to 15% of whites but is not found in Asians or blacks.

The gene codes for a protein called CCR5. This protein and another one called CXCR4 are located on the surface of a number of human cells. An article in the May 2003 edition of the *Journal of Virology* demonstrates that CCR5 and CXCR4 can be used as receptors by HIV-1 to enter and infect CD4+ T cells, dendritic cells, and macrophages. Furthermore, CCR5 was shown to be essential for viral transmission and replication during the early phase of the disease, even before symptoms of infection appear. Researchers anticipate that further investigation of the CCR5 gene will eventually help them to develop drugs to prevent or destroy HIV in newborns.

HIV-POSITIVE WOMEN HAVING BABIES

Many HIV-positive women who have babies are not aware of their HIV status. Even when pregnant women learn that they are HIV-positive they often decide to continue the pregnancy despite the risk of passing the infection to their babies. Some women choose to become pregnant already knowing that they are infected with

HIV. Many people consider HIV-positive women who decide to have babies to be selfish and unconcerned with the potentially tragic consequences of their actions. Still others regard the decision as strictly personal and understandable. The choice an HIV-positive woman makes to give birth can reflect an optimism that is fostered by effective drug therapies and a new reality—many people with HIV infection are living longer, more comfortably, and asymptomatically.

The choice to bear children also reflects societal and environmental realities, as well as attitudes about death and illness. Most women with HIV/AIDS live in poverty; they do not have easy access to medical care, and socio-economic problems such as violence, homelessness, separated families, and low literacy rates challenge children's chances of leading long, safe, and healthy lives. Tracie M. Gardner, an AIDS policy analyst for the Federation of Protestant Welfare Agencies, believes that for many women in poor communities HIV infection is the least of their problems. Gardner tells the story of a pregnant inner-city woman in her early twenties who, when told she was HIV infected and had ten years to live, replied that this was nine more years than she thought she had.

LIVING LONG ENOUGH TO KNOW
Surviving into Their Teens

When children who are fifteen to seventeen years old in the early 2000s were born, much less was known about HIV/AIDS. With increased understanding of the disease has come the development of strategies that are increasing the outlook for those infected with HIV. Officials at the CDC report that most children infected from birth now survive beyond age five. CDC statistics from 2001 indicate that 3,923 children (those children up to age twelve) in the United States were HIV-positive. While many HIV-infected children die as infants and toddlers, it is not uncommon for others to reach their teens.

Medical experts distinguish three distinct patterns of disease progression among HIV-infected children. The first group consists of approximately one-quarter of those infected who display symptoms within their first eighteen months following infection. Even with treatment, progression to AIDS in this group is more rapid than for the other two groups. Children in the second group experience a less aggressive progression and often have milder or less prolonged symptomatic periods of symptoms. These children tend to live to be about three to five years old. The third group is a recently emerging group of survivors. These children have grown up with few, if any, symptoms. Some were not diagnosed until they were nine to eleven years old. From New York City, where more than one-fifth of the nation's pediatric AIDS cases reside, there are reports of children as old as fourteen who were infected at birth but remained asymptomatic and undiagnosed. Researchers are understandably eager to determine why these children remain asymptomatic in spite of their infection.

Dealing with Physical and Emotional Problems

When HIV-infected children died in the early years of the AIDS epidemic, they were generally unaware of what was happening to them. Today, at the Children's Evaluation and Rehabilitation Center of the Albert Einstein College of Medicine's Rose Kennedy Center in the Bronx, school-aged children meet with social workers in a support group to handle the physical and emotional ordeals of growing up with HIV and AIDS. These children are part of the increasing number born with HIV who have survived long enough to realize what it means. They must learn to cope with the physical, psychological, and emotional consequences of HIV/AIDS.

HIV-positive children deal with problems unique to their situations—a mother's death from AIDS, keeping their disease a secret from classmates at school, the fear of dying, and coping with the deaths of members of their support group. Other concerns range from the dread of having their teeth pulled (because HIV-positive people's teeth decay unusually quickly) to the taunting the children receive at school because they may be short and underweight. Discussions range from what heaven is like to practical advice about taking ZDV in capsules rather than the bitter liquid form. When asked by a visitor what he wanted to be when he grew up, one child in a support group responded, "I never think about it."

One More Problem

Many children who are HIV-positive do not know it. In some cases their parents or foster parents have tried to protect them and do not want them to know. Others fear that the children will not be able to keep the news from other children, teachers, and neighbors. Some parents do not tell their children for fear the children will blame them for passing on the infection. Just as poignantly, many who do know keep their illness a secret even from their siblings. For those who know about their condition, HIV/AIDS is one more hardship in a life often made difficult by poverty, instability, and the loss of loved ones—especially parents. A child whose mother died from AIDS when he was five years old was understandably bitter about the fact that he was the only one of three siblings to be infected.

WHO WILL CARE FOR THEM?

The HIV/AIDS epidemic has created many tragedies, including millions of orphans. The World Health Organization in Geneva, Switzerland, estimates that by the end of 2000 there were more than thirteen million children worldwide orphaned by parents who died of AIDS. According to U.S. experts, forty million children worldwide will lose one or both parents to AIDS between 1997 and 2010. In Africa alone, during 1999 there were more than eight million AIDS orphans and one million HIV-positive children.

It is not always possible to find someone to care for an orphan of parents who died of AIDS, particularly if the child also has HIV or AIDS. Some family members may be hesitant to take in the child for fear he or she may spread the infection. In a growing number of cases, however, grandparents (in most cases, grandmothers) are taking these orphans into their homes. This may be a burden on older people who have lost their own children and may feel too old, tired, or impoverished to rear another family. They may also fear that they will die before their grandchildren do, leaving no one to care for them. It is no less difficult for the children who have lost their parents and fear they will probably miss the advantages they would have had with younger parents, such as being able to play more active childhood games.

Older orphans struggle with the rage, shame, and isolation of losing a parent to AIDS. Observers are finding that the AIDS epidemic is creating a class of particularly troubled youth. All children who lose a parent suffer to some degree, but for those whose parents die from AIDS, embarrassment and secrecy often compound the trauma. Teens whose parents became infected as a result of injecting drugs or practicing unsafe sex are often torn between feeling sorry for their parents and blaming them for their illnesses.

ADOLESCENTS, YOUNG ADULTS, AND HIV/AIDS
Patterns of Infection

The transmission and course of AIDS among adolescents and adults follow similar patterns. In 2003 male adults and adolescents were infected primarily as a result of male to male sexual activity (MTM; 48%), unidentified exposure (22%), or intravenous drug use (IDU; 15%). Female adults and adolescents, on the other hand, became infected through IDU (20%), unidentified activity (34%), or heterosexual contact (45%).

The characteristics of adolescence—a time of development, uncertainty, and a misleading sense of bravado and immortality, often combined with pushing the boundaries of good sense—create the potential for some young people to become particularly vulnerable to HIV infection. For many, this is a time of experimentation and risk-taking, often in terms of sexual behavior or use of alcohol and illicit drugs. Some adolescents, struggling with their sexuality, may engage in homosexual encounters away from home but maintain and engage in heterosexual relationships in their neighborhoods to avoid suspicion.

Clinics for Homeless and Runaway Youth.

In the early 1990s the CDC conducted anonymous surveys at clinics and shelters for homeless young people and runaways to gather information about risk behavior. Despite the anonymity of the surveys, the prevalence of certain behaviors, such as male to male sexual contact and intravenous drug use, were probably underreported because most teens are reluctant to admit to such behaviors. Nonetheless, the prevalence of recorded HIV risks was quite high.

Four to 28% of all male clients at four clinics for homeless and runaway youth had a history of MTM contact. This risk behavior accounted for 25 to 95% of all HIV infections among males at each clinic. Heterosexual women without a history of IDU accounted for 66 to 100% of the HIV infections among women, implying that infection came from contact with infected partners. Surprisingly, IDU was responsible for relatively few HIV infections; fewer than 2% of clients at three clinics and 17% at one clinic reported IDU. Only six of the 103 (6%) HIV-positive clients at the four clinics that conducted the risk surveys reported intravenous drug use.

Most Adolescents Are Sexually Active

Even though the growth rate of HIV/AIDS has slowed in the United States, the rate among young Americans continues to rise. Most HIV cases among youth have been spread sexually. According to the CDC, approximately three-fourths of adolescents who become infected with HIV are heterosexual females and adolescent males who engage in MTM.

Adolescents are having sex more frequently and earlier than ever before. According to the CDC, in 1999, 11.7% of ninth graders reported that they had engaged in sexual intercourse before the age of thirteen, and 38.6% of them revealed they had sexual intercourse by the ninth grade. In 1999, 65% of high school seniors reported that they had engaged in sexual intercourse.

Additionally, about one-fourth of teenagers (23%) also reported having had sex with four or more partners. Among sexually active students, fewer than half (46%) had used a latex condom during their last sexual intercourse.

SEXUALLY TRANSMITTED DISEASES. Teenagers engaging in sexual activity before becoming sufficiently mature, together with ineffective contraceptive methods, have led to record high rates of sexually transmitted diseases (STDs) among heterosexuals. Of the estimated twelve million new cases of STDs in the United States each year, three million (25%) occur among thirteen- to nineteen-years-olds. According to the CDC, about one out of five Americans twelve and older has an STD; most in this group are unaware they are infected.

Although overall rates of infection for some STDs, such as gonorrhea, declined during the 1990s, gonorrhea infections among African-Americans increased by more than 5% from 1997 to 1999, and infection with genital herpes also increased. The CDC publication "STD Surveillance 2003" reported that gonorrhea infection rates among African-Americans were twenty times higher than those among whites. More than one out of five Americans is estimated to have genital herpes infection, with teenage African-American women being especially vulnerable.

Studies and health education programs in the early 2000s have focused on teaching African-American teens ages fourteen to eighteen about the relationship between consistent condom use and the prevention of STDs. But condoms are less effective in halting the spread of genital herpes than other STDs because herpes may be transmitted from parts of the body not covered by a condom.

LEADING THE WAY: YOUNG PEOPLE AS AIDS ACTIVISTS AND ORGANIZATIONS THAT HELP YOUNG PATIENTS

Almost since the beginning of the epidemic, children and teenagers have been among the activists campaigning for HIV/AIDS reforms and awareness of the disease. Their role has been a profoundly personal one. For example, until his death from AIDS on April 8, 1990, Ryan White—an Indiana teenager—generated worldwide attention to the disease and, in particular, to the stigmas and misconceptions surrounding it. White, who contracted the virus during treatment for his hemophilia, was a white, middle-class heterosexual boy, which ran counter to public perception at the time of AIDS as a disease of gay men.

Being expelled from school because of the supposed health risk to other students galvanized White to educate others on the nature of HIV and AIDS. His legacy includes the Ryan White Comprehensive AIDS Resources Emergency (CARE) Act, the multi-billion-dollar program that funds programs to help provide primary health care and support to those living with HIV/AIDS. As of 2005 the $2.1 billion Act is under threat due to federal government budget cuts.

An organization called AIDS Alliance for Children, Youth & Families (www.aids-alliance.org/aids_alliance/index.html) was established in 1994 to publicize the concerns of women, children, young people, and families who are affected by HIV/AIDS. The nonprofit organization is also a clearinghouse for relevant information and advocates for public policy changes in the areas of HIV/AIDS social welfare and disease prevention.

The National Association of People with AIDS (www.napwa.org), founded in 1993, advocates for people, including children, who live with HIV/AIDS. The nonprofit organization—the oldest national AIDS organizations in the United States—is a strong advocate for HIV/AIDS social programs and research funding.

MetroTeenAIDS (www.metroteenaids.org) is a Washington, D.C.-based organization that focuses on prevention, education, and treatment needs of teenagers. Through its Web site and in-person contact at schools, nightclubs, youth centers, shelters, and on the street, MetroTeenAIDS connects with teenagers in language that is relevant to them. The intent is to help teenagers protect themselves from the risks of HIV exposure and contamination, and in securing medical care for HIV infection and AIDS.

MetroTeenAIDS has been working in conjunction with numerous other youth and AIDS activists groups since 1994 to host annual conferences around the country that focus on educating young people about HIV and AIDS. In 1995 the conference became known as the Ryan White National Youth Conference on HIV and AIDS (RWNYC). In 2001 the first Positive Youth Institute—a one-day gathering specifically focusing on the needs of HIV-positive young people—was held prior to and in conjunction with the RWNYC. Each year approximately six hundred young people, health care workers, and AIDS activists attend the Conference (http://www.rwnyc.org/overview.htm).

CHAPTER 6
HIV/AIDS COSTS AND TREATMENT

FINANCING HEALTH CARE DELIVERY

Care for HIV/AIDS patients is expensive. Newer drug treatments, most prominently highly active antiretroviral therapy (HAART), have high per-unit costs. Nonetheless, their introduction in 1996 reduced total health care spending on AIDS by reducing the rate of hospitalization and use of outpatient care. According to a study conducted by the Rand Corporation and published in the March 15, 2001, issue of the *New England Journal of Medicine*, the average HIV patient incurred costs of about $1,410 per month in 1998. Extended over the full year, a patient's drug treatment for HIV could cost as much as $18,000. People with AIDS could spend up to $77,000 a year on treatment.

Longer survival periods following an AIDS diagnosis lead to even greater costs for care and treatment. For example, according to statistics from New York City released in an August 11, 2005, report from the Independent Budget Office, Department of Health and Mental Hygiene, the average survival time of AIDS patients in that city increased from five months in 1981 to eighty-two months in 2003.

Figures from the same report, published in the August 11, 2005, issue of *Newsday*, illustrate the effects of the increasing treatment costs and enhanced survival. The amount spent by the city's HIV/AIDS Services Administration rose from $117 million in fiscal year 1999 to $193 million in fiscal year 2004.

Some HIV/AIDS patients rely on health insurance to help pay these costs. But many patients are not insured. And many policies exclude or deny coverage to people with preexisting conditions, and, as a result, many HIV-positive people are denied private health insurance.

According to the Office of National AIDS Policy, a White House agency, approximately half of all adults and nearly 90% of children living with HIV/AIDS in the United States have the costs of their treatment paid for by Medicaid. Medicaid is an entitlement program run by state and federal governments to provide health care insurance to patients younger than sixty-five who cannot afford to pay for private health insurance. Medicaid eligibility requirements vary from state to state. Generally, however, the program covers people with incomes of less than $700 per month who cannot support themselves financially due to a physical or mental impairment—an impairment that is expected to last at least one year or result in death. The operation of Medicaid programs also varies widely by jurisdiction. Many states supplement federal funding with their own funds, and each state determines its eligibility criteria and benefits—the number and type of treatments provided through the program.

The toll of AIDS on the Medicaid program is huge. For example, during 2004 the Medicaid program paid for services for an estimated 195,000 people living with AIDS at a cost of $5.4 billion. Between 1986 and 2000 the number of people living with AIDS who received Medicaid benefits increased by about 215%, and Medicaid expenditures increased by more than 1,860%. For example, in fiscal year 1995 Medicaid spending for HIV/AIDS care was $1.5 billion. In fiscal year 2003 it had risen to $8.5 billion, according to the Centers for Medicare and Medicaid Services.

A Reverse in Federal Policy

In early 1997 the administration of President Bill Clinton announced that it hoped to expand Medicaid to cover all low-income HIV-infected people. The administration had hoped to give low-income HIV-positive people access to HAART drugs that slow the onset of AIDS. By the end of the year, however, the administration announced that it could not follow through because such a nationwide plan would increase government spending. Both the Clinton administration and the administrations of George W. Bush forbade the federal government and states to change the Medicaid rules if that change would increase spending over a five-year period. As of 2005, only patients who have been diagnosed with AIDS, not those who are HIV-positive, are covered by Medicaid.

Domestic spending cuts announced by President George W. Bush in February 2005 included trimming $45 to 60 billion from the Medicaid budget over the next ten years, which will further limit the number of AIDS patients who receive treatment through Medicaid.

State Programs to Provide Drugs

In the late 1980s state-administered programs were established to help AIDS patients pay for azidothymidine (now called zidovudine, or ZDV), the newest effective drug at the time. The programs give free drugs to AIDS patients who are not poor enough to qualify for Medicaid coverage but who do not have private health insurance coverage, or patients who have used up their prescription drug coverage. The federal government provides two-thirds of the funding for the state programs, and the balance comes mostly from the states. In fiscal year 1996 federal and state drug program expenditures totaled about $145 million. These costs have risen dramatically. For example, Medicaid expenditures for HIV antiretroviral drugs in fiscal year 2003 were approximately $630 million.

Until recently, these programs did not attract many participants, primarily because ZDV alone was not very effective against the disease. In the late 1990s, however, with the development of a new class of antiretroviral drugs—called protease inhibitors (PIs)—that seem to reduce the amount of virus in the blood, more patients wanted to take advantage of the programs. (The typical three-drug "cocktail"—one new PI combined with two other HIV/AIDS medications—costs at least $12,000 per year per patient.)

This growing demand has put a financial strain on the programs, and many states have to ration HIV/AIDS drugs or turn patients away in order to remain solvent. Some states are making it harder for people to qualify for the programs, and a few are beginning to charge small copayments (a percentage of the total cost that the patient is responsible for paying) to offset the cost of the drugs. Several states do not offer the new drugs through their programs. More than thirty states offer at least one PI, but seventeen states do not provide any. Even after cutbacks in their AIDS drug programs, some states may run out of money before they receive more federal funds.

By 2004 the number of uninsured people with HIV and AIDS who were on waiting lists for state AIDS Drug Assistance Programs (ADAPs) had climbed into the thousands. North Carolina had the nation's longest waiting list, at 940 people. Among the states with waiting lists were Alabama, Alaska, Idaho, Iowa, Kentucky, Montana, South Dakota, and West Virginia.

ADAPs, which operate in all fifty states, provide medications to approximately 136,000 people each year. But funding is state-controlled and discretionary. This can lead to capping the enrollment of eligible people in the program, as was done in 2004 in Utah, Arizona, and Indiana, or reducing the funds provided for aid, as was done in 2004 in Idaho and in 2005 in Massachusetts, Nebraska, New Hampshire, New Jersey, and Oregon.

Costs to the Insurance Industry

Some employers, largely those that are self-insured and paying premiums to third-party insurers as protection against catastrophic health care claims, have put caps on expenditures for HIV/AIDS treatments. In some cases these employers have reduced their policies from million-dollar lifetime coverage to $10,000, which does not cover a year's worth of treatment. Because self-insured plans are exempt from most states' insurance regulations, employees covered by such plans who acquire HIV have no protection from insurance caps.

NEW LIFE INSURANCE AVAILABLE. In 1997 Guarantee Trust Life Insurance Company, a small Midwestern company, began to offer life insurance to some HIV-positive people. Company president Richard S. Holson III said the company decided to offer the coverage because it believes that many HIV-positive people are otherwise healthy and should be viewed as having a treatable chronic illness rather than a terminal disease. With new treatments available, affected people are living longer.

The policies provide up to $250,000 coverage and are offered to those who acquired the virus through sexual activity or accidental needle sticks. Applicants must be between the ages of twenty-one and forty-nine, have previous and current CD4 tests of 400 or greater, and never have been diagnosed with AIDS. Coverage is not offered to people who acquired the disease through the injection of drugs because drug use increases the company's risks, including the chance that prescribed medications will not be taken. The coverage is expensive: a typical thirty-year-old nonsmoking male who is HIV-positive pays $1,500 per month for the $250,000 policy.

Following this lead, Dutch insurance companies are poised to begin offering life insurance policies to some people infected with HIV. The Union of Insurers in the Netherlands, which represents more than 80% of the Dutch market, has decided to begin offering coverage in 2005. Coverage will be offered to those who have responded positively to treatment with antiretroviral drugs.

Changes to the Health Care System

Since the 1960s U.S. government spending on health services has consistently increased. Federal health expenses rose from 15% of the federal budget in 1990 to 20% in 2005. At the same time health care providers—doctors, hospitals, and other health-related institutions and professions—have watched as payments for Medicare, Medicaid, and private insurance coverage, once easily obtained in the 1960s and 1970s, were increasingly laden with restrictions and limits. In the 1990s providers also encountered a greater resistance among private insurers to pay. Bureaucratic management, increasing amounts of paperwork to document medical care and claims, and slow reimbursement rates prompted some physicians to stop caring for Medicare/Medicaid patients. Managed-care programs, which often restrict physicians' professional decisions and patient choices, were initially designed to control medical care costs.

As of 2005 many managed-care programs, also known as health maintenance organizations (HMOs) and preferred provider organizations (PPOs), are having administrative and financial problems. These programs, which rely heavily on primary care practitioners (general and family physicians), are shifting the focus of treatment they provide for HIV/AIDS patients. Beginning around the year 2000, a large number of HIV-infected people enrolled in managed-care networks. This is in part because more companies are placing all employees in HMOs and PPOs, and in part because government insurance programs are also directing Medicaid recipients to such programs.

A NEW MANAGED-CARE PROGRAM FOR HIV/AIDS PATIENTS: THE TENNESSEE "CENTERS OF EXCELLENCE" PROGRAM. On January 1, 1994, Tennessee withdrew from the federal Medicaid program and began to implement a state health care reform plan called Tennessee Medicaid (TennCare). In May 1998 TennCare introduced a voluntary managed-care program for its members with HIV or AIDS. The model program features "Centers of Excellence" providers—practitioners with high levels of expertise in the care of HIV/AIDS patients. The providers must agree to adopt and adhere to a clinical protocol (set of rules) developed by a committee composed of providers, consumers, managed-care organizations, and public health officials. The protocol committee meets up to twice a month to discuss and recommend new drug therapies as they become available and to inform participating providers about new treatments.

Providers may be individual practitioners with access to needed services or full-service clinics composed of a group of practitioners. There are no financial incentives to participate in the program. However, providers who meet the Centers of Excellence criteria do not have to obtain prior authorization when they prescribe drugs or treatments that fall under the clinical protocols.

The Centers of Excellence program frees managed-care organizations (MCOs) from the clinical and administrative responsibility of keeping close tabs on HIV and AIDS care. It also allows MCOs to remain confident that providers are capable and have access to a wide range of services needed by members. MCO members know that participating providers meet high standards of HIV/AIDS clinical care. Other managed care programs are developing comparable programs to meet the unique health and social service needs of people living with HIV/AIDS.

The program, which costs $5.1 billion a year, has endured criticism since its beginning. Doctors and hospitals have complained that it has been underfunded, forcing them to carry an unfair proportion of the costs. But despite its rocky history, TennCare was renewed on July 1, 2002, in a five-year agreement with the federal government.

CHALLENGES FOR THE DELIVERY SYSTEM

HIV/AIDS poses a major challenge to health care institutions, health care professionals, and others who provide direct health care services. HIV/AIDS is a relatively new disease, whereas most medical knowledge is acquired over many years or generations. The health care system cares for about one million people in the United States suffering from a disease that is still only partly understood. The system must also plan to deliver services to the tens of thousands of people in the United States who are HIV-positive and will require specialized health care services during the coming years, although only a small proportion will need intensive medical care at any one time.

The number of indigent people in need of HIV/AIDS care, particularly those who bring the added complications of drug addiction, homelessness, and other socioeconomic problems, has strained public hospitals in particular. Patients in public hospitals are often different from those in private hospitals. They generally seek care later in the course of the disease's progression and are, therefore, sicker. The scarcity of resources—trained personnel, hospital beds, and support services—in the community, combined with inadequate funding and reimbursement for HIV/AIDS care, are significant obstacles to effective health care delivery for poor HIV/AIDS patients.

Office Visits

Some physicians, particularly those who handle many HIV/AIDS patients, have extended their office hours or hired counselors to deal with these patients because their visits are time-consuming. Physicians polled by the Centers for Disease Control and Prevention

TABLE 6.1

Number and percent of office visits, by diagnostic/screening services ordered or provided and patient's sex, 2000

Diagnostic and screening services ordered or provided	Number of visits in thousands[a]	Percent of visits	Female[b] Percent of visits	Male[c] Percent of visits
All visits	823,542	. . .	. . .	. . .
None	210,404	25.5	23.6	28.4
Examinations				
Skin	87,837	10.7	10.6	10.8
Visual	59,923	7.3	6.8	7.9
Pelvic	59,062	7.21	1.0	*1.6
Breast	57,041	6.9	10.7	*1.5
Rectal	42,683	5.2	5.0	5.5
Glaucoma	24,593	3.0	3.1	2.8
Hearing	16,785	2.0	1.5	2.8
Tests				
Blood pressure	373,429	45.3	48.5	40.8
Urinalysis	79,970	9.71	1.1	7.7
Hematocrit/hemoglobin	42,925	5.2	5.5	4.8
Cholesterol	39,608	4.8	4.4	5.5
Pap test	29,952	3.6	6.1	*
EKG[d]	22,937	2.8	2.2	3.6
PSA[e]	12,514	1.5	*	3.7
Strep test	11,287	1.4	1.6	1.1
Pregnancy test	5,392	0.7	1.1	*
Blood lead level	2,687	0.3	*0.3	*
HIV serology[f]	2,560	0.3	0.4	*
Other STD[g]	3,793	0.5	0.7	*
Other blood test	113,572	13.8	14.4	12.8
Imaging				
X ray	53,419	6.5	5.6	7.8
Ultrasound	20,054	2.4	3.0	1.7
Mammography	17,836	2.2	3.7	*
CAT scan/MRI[h,i]	13,232	1.6	1.6	1.6
Other	118,017	14.3	13.9	14.9
Blank	10,303	1.3	1.0	1.6

Note: . . .Category not applicable.
*Figure does not meet standard of reliability or precision.
[a]Total exceeds "All visits" because more than one service may be reported per visit.
[b]Based on 488,199,000 visits made by females.
[c]Based on 335,343,000 visits made by males.
[d]EKG is electrocardiogram.
[e]PSA is prostate-specific antigen.
[f]HIV is human immunodeficiency virus.
[g]STD is sexually transmitted disease.
[h]CAT is computerized axial tomography.
[i]MRI is magnetic resonance imaging.

SOURCE: Donald K. Cherry and David A. Woodwell, "Table 15. Number and Percent of Office Visits with Corresponding Standard Errors, by Diagnostic and Screening Services Ordered or Provided and Patient's Sex, 2000," in "National Ambulatory Medical Care Survey: 2000 Summary," in *Advance Data From Vitaland Health Statistics*, no. 328, June 5, 2002

TABLE 6.2

Number and percent of office visits, by therapeutic/preventative services ordered or provided and patient's sex, 2000

Therapeutic and preventive services ordered or provided	Number of visits in thousands[a]	Percent of visits	Female[b] Percent of visits	Male[c] Percent of visits
All visits	823,542	. . .	. . .	. . .
None	515,550	62.6	61.6	64.0
Counseling/education				
Diet	126,988	15.4	15.4	15.5
Exercise	80,839	9.8	9.8	9.8
Injury prevention	24,610	3.0	2.5	3.6
Growth/development	21,460	2.6	2.2	3.2
Stress management	18,403	2.2	2.5	1.8
Prenatal instructions	18,396	2.2	3.8	*
Mental health	18,221	2.2	2.2	2.2
Tobacco use/exposure	18,213	2.2	2.0	2.5
Breast self-examination	17,827	2.2	3.6	*
Skin cancer prevention	14,311	1.7	1.4	2.2
Family planning/contraception	9,564	1.2	1.9	*
HIV/STD transmission[d,e]	5,190	0.6	0.9	0.3
Other therapy				
Complementary and alternative medicine	31,589	3.8	3.8	3.9
Physiotherapy	22,273	2.7	2.5	2.9
Psycho-pharmacotherapy	19,947	2.4	2.3	2.6
Psychotherapy	18,669	2.3	2.2	2.4
Other	36,839	4.5	4.3	4.7
Blank	21,356	2.6	2.3	3.0

Note: . . . Category not applicable.
*Figure does not meet standard of reliability or precision.
[a]Total exceeds "All visits" because more than one service may be reported per visit.
[b]Based on 488,199,000 visits made by females.
[c]Based on 335,343,000 made by males.
[d]HIV is human immunodeficiency virus.
[e]STD is sexually transmitted disease.

SOURCE: "Table 16. Number and Percent of Office Visits with Corresponding Standard Errors, by Therapeutic and Preventative Services Ordered or Provided and Patient's Sex, 2000," in "National Ambulatory Medical Care Survey: 2000 Summary," in *Advance Data From Vital and Health Statistics*, no. 328, June 5, 2002

(CDC) reported more than 2.5 million patient visits for HIV in 2000. (See Table 6.1.) While this represented only about 0.3% of the estimated 824 million visits for all causes in 2000, it did not reflect the growing amount of time spent on diagnostic and screening services in each office or the increase in the number of visits devoted to counseling and educating HIV/AIDS patients. According to the same survey, 5.2 million office visits provided counseling for and education about HIV and sexually transmitted disease transmission (0.6% of all patient visits). (See Table 6.2.)

Hospital Care

The nation's approximately seven thousand hospitals are also feeling the pinch of Medicare rate limits, reduced payments from MCOs, and intense competition from other providers, such as ambulatory surgical centers and hospices. Many are struggling to remain profitable institutions. During the 1970s and 1980s the steady growth of "for-profit" hospitals lured many privately insured, middle-class patients away from community hospitals, leaving most of the uninsured, sicker patients to seek care from inner-city public hospitals.

Most HIV/AIDS patients are cared for in inner-city public hospitals that are already overburdened with inadequate revenues, staff shortages, lack of referral facilities, and emergency rooms used by many poor neighborhood residents as sources of primary medical care. Many health care professionals praise San Francisco's model of care. This California city was hit hard in the early days of the epidemic and developed a range of innovative, effective programs in response to acute need during the early 1990s. This model of care relies on extensive outpatient services and volunteer social support services provided by the well-established and well-organized gay and lesbian community.

Changes in Health Care Delivery

Although fewer people are acquiring HIV/AIDS, the evolution of HIV care is altering the ways in which health care is delivered. In the late stages of AIDS most patients require intermittent hospitalization and home health care. Those who are not as severely affected and have symptoms or conditions that once required intravenous therapy (which had to be administered in a hospital or by home health professionals) are now able to self-medicate at home. Many drugs are now available for oral administration in pill or liquid form. These home care and community-based measures lessen the burden on the health care delivery system and make it easier for HIV/AIDS patients to care for themselves.

People with AIDS (PWAs) who receive informal home health care (such as care from friends and family) often use fewer hospital services, perhaps reflecting a greater desire to remain at home. PWAs with strong social support systems and who prefer to remain at home may also be less likely to demand an aggressive approach to treating their illness. Those who receive formal home health care (visits from physicians, nurses, therapists, social workers, case managers, and other paid caregivers) often use more hospital services. This may reflect a greater use of all types of health services by PWAs with weaker social support systems and/or an aggressive approach to treatment by medical professionals.

An AIDS Care Alternative

In 1993, in an effort to offer Atlanta's 4,400 uninsured AIDS patients treatment equal to that available to patients with private insurance, Grady Memorial Hospital opened a $7 million outpatient HIV/AIDS clinic. Since that time the clinic and its 150-member staff have provided emergency care, dental services, mental health counseling, social and support services, HIV research and education, case management, and babysitting. The clinic is partially financed under a provision of the Ryan White Comprehensive AIDS Resources Emergency (CARE) Act of 1990 (PL 101–381), which was enacted to provide funding to improve the quality and availability of care for HIV-infected people. In 1994 the clinic began asking patients to pay nominal fees based on their incomes. Under the CARE Act, providers may charge up to 10% of a patient's wages.

Hospice Care

The AIDS epidemic has had a significant impact on hospices. Hospice care, both in the home and in special-ized centers, offers care aimed at comfort rather than cure. This includes expert pain relief, along with emotional, psychological, and spiritual support for patients, their families, and friends. The majority of hospice patients are older adults who suffer from terminal diseases such as cancer and face imminent death.

At the beginning of the AIDS epidemic patients did not fit well into the hospices of the day. AIDS patients were younger than traditional hospice patients, and the progression of their disease was less predictable than many cancers. Furthermore, as one hospice administrator noted, because many people with AIDS were accustomed to prejudice, they initially mistrusted the motivation and altruism of hospice workers. In the early 2000s, more than two decades after the first cases of AIDS were identified, home-based hospice programs designed to meet the needs of AIDS patients, their partners, and families have gained acceptance in the medical community as well as among HIV-infected people and the voluntary social service agencies organized to support them.

HEALTH CARE PROVIDERS

Physicians

AIDS physicians have been defined as doctors who perform a wide variety of services in addition to providing care to AIDS patients. Many are also AIDS activists and may be involved in developing policies, planning for care needs, and dealing with the media.

One challenge in the training of physicians to treat AIDS patients is that AIDS care requires skills and training in the multitude of conditions known to be part of HIV/AIDS. However, the amount of experience—rather than the kind of training—may be a better predictor of the quality of care the physician is able to deliver.

A 1996 study headed by M. M. Kitahata, published in the *New England Journal of Medicine* (vol. 334), claims that AIDS patients treated by primary care physicians with no previous experience dealing with the disease died more than a year earlier than those whose doctors had treated at least five AIDS patients. The study also shows that patients had a 46% decrease in relative risk of death at any given time when treated by a physician who had treated other AIDS patients. The difference, according to the researchers, was that the more experienced physicians consulted more frequently with specialists and reported more visits with their AIDS patients. Since that time, the study's findings have been verified by further research (W. E. Cunningham et al., "The Effect of Hospital Experience on Mortality among Patients Hospitalized with Acquired Immunodeficiency Syndrome in California," *American Journal of Medicine*, vol. 107, no. 2, August 1999; M. M. Kitahata et al., "Primary Care Delivery Is Associated with Greater

Physician Experience and Improved Survival among Persons with AIDS," *Journal of General Internal Medicine*, vol. 18, no. 2, 2003).

MORE PHYSICIANS ARE WILLING TO TREAT HIV PATIENTS. The AIDS epidemic began at a time when many newly graduated physicians were not choosing primary care specialties such as internal medicine, the most fitting for the ongoing care required by HIV-infected patients. Some observers feared that new physicians would avoid practicing in geographic areas where there were large proportions of HIV/AIDS patients.

Fortunately, the CDC finds that most primary care doctors believe that they have an obligation to care for HIV-infected patients and are interested in further professional training to help increase their skill and comfort in caring for HIV/AIDS patients. Among physicians who report they do not provide care to AIDS patients, the majority cite a lack of experience with HIV and note that providers with more expertise are readily available in their communities.

Nurses

The impact of HIV/AIDS on nurses can be more difficult to assess than its effect on doctors. Nurses often have different viewpoints than some physicians about their professional obligations to patients with HIV. As hospital employees, nurses seldom have the option of choosing whether to treat a particular patient (nor do patients have much choice of nurses). Nurses, however, report that caring for HIV/AIDS patients can take an enormous emotional toll since they are often the primary source of continuous physical and emotional care for these patients, who generally require more care and services than other patients.

Nurses, physicians, and other health care professionals must cope with more than simply their fears of contracting the disease from HIV/AIDS patients and keeping abreast of advances in the treatment of the disease. They also face a wide range of emotional issues when caring for these patients, from feelings of failure when treatment is unsuccessful to grief when witnessing the untimely deaths of patients. Support groups and counselors help many health professionals, especially hospice workers, to share and understand these feelings so they are better able to care for HIV/AIDS patients and their families.

CDC Guidelines

In 1992, in response to an incident in which five patients acquired HIV from a Florida dentist, the CDC addressed occupational exposure to blood-borne pathogens. The CDC offered new guidelines to prevent the accidental spread of the infection from health care providers to patients and from patients to health care workers.

The recommendations stressed the careful and consistent use, with all patients, of standard infection control procedures for blood-borne agents—the so-called universal precautions—that were published by the CDC in 1987.

The CDC guidelines also recommended that HIV-infected health care workers stop performing what were termed "exposure-prone invasive procedures" and that professional medical and dental groups draw up lists of "exposure-prone procedures" for their disciplines. The CDC recommended that HIV-infected health care workers consult with a panel of experts to determine which, if any, limits should be placed on their medical practices and further advised practitioners to inform patients of their HIV-infection status before performing medical procedures.

The CDC guidelines resulted in some unforeseen consequences. Professional groups, hospital attorneys, state courts, legislatures, and the U.S. Congress reacted with alarm to a perception of dangers to patients posed by HIV-infected health care professionals totally out of proportion to the largely theoretical risk. According to the U.S. Public Health Service, the average risk of HIV infection after skin contact with HIV-infected blood is estimated to be about 0.3%, and the risk for transmission is probably even lower from contact with body fluids or tissues other than blood. Through 1990, forty cases of occupationally acquired HIV were documented. By the end of 2001 fifty-seven documented cases had been reported and 138 additional cases of HIV infection may be linked to occupational exposures (see below).

Most medical professional associations refused to cooperate in developing a list of exposure-prone invasive procedures that carry a higher risk of virus transmission. They did not believe there was enough data to support drawing up such a list. Nonetheless, the CDC did not withdraw its recommendation concerning the exposure-prone procedures list, even after studies of more than fifteen thousand patients cared for by thirty-two health care workers known to be HIV infected found that none of the patients contracted HIV as a result of the care.

The CDC also recommended that the following procedures and philosophies would best serve patients and health care workers:

- The universal and meticulous use of well-understood infection-control procedures, particularly those developed from the study of hepatitis B—another blood-borne infection that is one hundred times more infectious and ten times more common in health professionals—should be applied in all health care settings, whether hospital, office, or home based.

- Operative or other invasive procedures, in which injury to health care professionals occurs with any frequency, should be discontinued or modified to the greatest extent possible. This involves developing new instruments and investigating new operative techniques.

- All health care professionals should consider being tested for HIV. An HIV-positive result, however, should not justify restricting the practice of health care professionals.

The National Commission on AIDS did not agree with all of the CDC guidelines, cautioning against placing too much emphasis on HIV transmission in health care settings. Unwarranted emphasis in the wrong place, the commission noted, distracts the nation from proper attention to sexual transmission, transmission via intravenous drug use, the problems of sexually active teenagers, and an epidemic that needs more committed health care professionals.

The commission also warned that the costs associated with testing all health care professionals and all patients would amount to $1.5 billion and that there was no evidence that such testing would increase patient or worker safety.

Should Doctors Tell Patients?

Since 1991 the American College of Surgeons (ACS), the nation's largest professional organization of surgeons, has, in defiance of CDC guidelines, refused to draw up a list of procedures that might pose a high risk of transmitting HIV from doctor to patient. The group maintains that since not a single documented case of surgeon-to-patient transmission has been established, there is no scientific basis for suggesting that a particular surgical procedure increases the risk of viral transmission. The ACS also notes that surgical patients are at greater risk for other surgery-related infections than for HIV, even from an HIV-infected physician.

The CDC guidelines, published in the July 12, 1991, issue of *Mortality and Morbidity Weekly Report* ("Recommendations for Preventing Transmission of Human Immunodeficiency Virus and Hepatitis B Virus to Patients during Exposure-Prone Invasive Procedures"), instruct HIV-infected health care workers to avoid contact with patients that could potentially bring the worker's blood into contact with a patient's body cavities or mucous membranes.

HEALTH CARE WORKERS AND INFECTION

Health Care Workers with HIV and AIDS

As of December 2003 the CDC was aware of only fifty-seven documented cases of health care workers other than surgeons in the United States who had become infected with HIV as a result of occupational exposures. The breakdown of those who were infected was as follows: nurses (twenty-four), clinical laboratory workers (sixteen), nonsurgical physicians (six), nonclinical laboratory technicians (three), housekeeper/maintenance workers (two), surgical technicians (two), embalmer/morgue technician (one), health aide/attendant (one), respiratory therapist (one), and dialysis technician (one).

The CDC was also aware of 138 cases of HIV infection or AIDS possibly linked to occupational exposure among health care workers as of December 2003. These workers have not reported other risk factors for HIV infection. They had reported a history of occupational exposure to blood, body fluids, or HIV-infected laboratory material but had not documented infection after a specific exposure.

The known and possible cases of occupational acquisition of HIV undoubtedly represent an underestimate. There are surely unknown numbers of people who acquired their infection through occupational exposures, although, even in 2005, this is conjectural.

As of 2005 twenty-one states had enacted needle-safety legislation to safeguard health care workers from blood-borne pathogen (agents that cause disease) exposures. State laws aim to strengthen and supplement the federal standards mandated by the Occupational Safety and Health Administration. Many of the state laws require the creation of a written exposure plan that is periodically reviewed and updated; protocols for safety device identification and selection; logs to document and report injuries with sharp instruments; and strict requirements and training for workers on how to use safety devices.

In 2001 the Public Health Service updated guidelines for treatment to prevent health care workers with occupational exposure to HIV from becoming infected with the virus. Known as "postexposure prophylaxis" (PEP), the recommendation is that affected workers be given a four-week regimen of two antiretroviral drugs such as zidovudine and lamivudine, with the addition of a third drug for HIV exposures that pose an increased risk of transmission. While the best strategy to protect health care workers is to avoid exposure to HIV and other blood-borne pathogens, PEP has, as of 2005, proven effective in preventing HIV infection in workers who have been exposed.

Risks to Patients

Health care officials are not the only ones worried about HIV transmission in the health care setting. Patients also fear that infected health care workers could transmit the virus to them. The CDC developed a model of the risk of HIV transmission to patients, estimating that the risk of a patient becoming infected by an HIV-positive surgeon during a single operation is anywhere from one in 42,000 to one in 420,000. This risk is considerably less than the risks associated with many other medical procedures.

Ongoing studies by the CDC of more than 15,700 patients of thirty-two HIV-infected health care workers found no documented evidence that HIV infections found in these studies could be attributed to medical or dental care, with the exception of the five patients of a Florida dentist in 1990. Medical researchers have tried without success to determine how the dentist infected his patients and whether the exposure was accidental or deliberate. One theory is that he did not properly sterilize his dental tools; another is that he accidentally cut his finger or jabbed himself with a hypodermic needle, did not notice it, and bled into the patients' mouths. Prior to his death in 1990, the dentist denied intentionally exposing his patients.

In 1990 Rudolph Almarez, a Baltimore breast surgeon who performed operations on as many as two thousand patients, died from AIDS. The nature of his death stirred up such concern that shortly after he died a Baltimore law firm solicited clients to seek legal advice, whether they were infected or not. The law firm told clients that they might be reimbursed for the emotional distress they now suffered if they sued the hospital where Almarez had practiced. Two separate legal complaints based on the fear of HIV exposure were dismissed by a Baltimore judge. The judge further stated that there were no allegations that Almarez had not followed recommended safety procedures or that any accident had taken place during surgery. None of the patients alleged infection from Almarez. A later study failed to find any HIV-positive patients among those Almarez had treated (*Rossi v. Almarez*, *Faya v. Almarez*, Baltimore City Cir. Ct. Nos. 90344028 CL123396; 90345011 CL12345g, May 23, 1991).

WHAT DOES IT COST TO TREAT HIV/AIDS PATIENTS?

In 2004 all federal government spending for HIV-related activities exceeded $16 billion. Federal spending for HIV/AIDS care alone totaled $11 billion. A full-scale clinical trial for a new drug costs between $9 and 18 million. The per-patient cost of HIV/AIDS drugs is between $12,000 and $70,000 a year depending on the severity of the patient's condition. Costs are expected to increase due to the rising costs of hospitalization, home care, insurance premiums and copayments, and physician services. Additionally, federal and state programs such as Medicaid have been forced to operate under tighter budgets and have eliminated certain treatments from insurance coverage. In 2000 certain drugs (including Bristol-Myers Squibb's enteric-coated formulation of didanosine and Abbott Laboratories' protease inhibitor ABT-378) rose substantially in price. Since then, concern over the rising price led to a self-imposed freeze in

pricing by some manufacturers in 2002. But in February 2003 Roche Pharmaceuticals announced that the price for Fuzeon, at the time the most expensive AIDS treatment on the market, will more than double in Europe.

Some expenses, however, have actually been reduced by relocating services from the hospital to a variety of outpatient settings. Examples of cost-saving services include outpatient transfusions and outpatient treatment for opportunistic infections such as *Pneumocystis carinii* pneumonia and cryptococcal meningitis. Increased volunteer-based social service programs that enable patients to be cared for at home also can prevent expensive hospital stays.

Federal government spending on HIV-related care and activities has increased steadily since 1985, when about $2 million was spent. In 2003 the budget office of the U.S. Public Health Service estimated that federal spending for HIV-related expenses was $16.7 billion, $10.2 billion of which was spent on medical care. Other government costs included research ($2.8 billion), education and prevention ($1.9 billion), and cash assistance ($1.7 billion), which is provided through the Social Security Administration and the Department of Housing and Urban Development. (See Table 6.3.)

The Ryan White Comprehensive AIDS Resources Emergency Act

In 1998 the Ryan White Comprehensive AIDS Resources Emergency (CARE) Act (PL 101–381) was the only federal program providing funds specifically for medical and support services to individuals with HIV and AIDS. The Act was named after Ryan White, who died of AIDS in 1990. White was an Indiana teenager with hemophilia who became infected through a blood transfusion. Shunned by his community because many people feared becoming infected through any kind of contact with him, White fought to attend school and attain rights for those infected with HIV/AIDS. White's efforts helped change the way the world treated those with the disease. The CARE Act was signed in 1990 and reauthorized in 1996 and 2000. The 2000 reauthorization addressed additional initiatives including improving access to care for vulnerable populations (such as women, minorities, and those with addictions or mental health disorders), increased accountability of providers, and improving services in underserved rural and urban regions.

CARE Act funds are appropriated using four formulas (Titles I–IV). The Title I formula provides emergency assistance to metropolitan areas disproportionately affected by the HIV epidemic. To qualify for Title I funds, eligible metropolitan areas (EMAs) must have more than two thousand cumulative AIDS cases reported during the preceding five years and a population of at least five hundred thousand. (The population provision

TABLE 6.3

Federal spending for HIV-related activities, according to agency and type of activity, selected years 1985–2003

[Data are compiled from federal government appropriations]

Agency and type of activity	1985	1990	1995	1999	2000	2001	2002[a]	2003
Agency				**Amount in millions**				
All federal spending	$209	$3,070	$7,019	$10,779	$12,025	$14,184	$14,988	$16,677
Department of Health and Human Services, total	201	2,372	5,200	8,494	9,621	11,406	12,039	13,292
Department of Health and Human Services discretionary spending, total[b]	109	1,592	2,700	4,094	4,546	5,226	5,789	6,142
National Institutes of Health	66	908	1,334	1,793	2,004	2,247	2,499	2,717
Substance Abuse and Mental Health Services Administration	—	50	24	92	110	157	169	171
Centers for Disease Control and Prevention	33	443	590	657	687	859	931	936
Food and Drug Administration	9	57	73	70	76	76	76	80
Health Resources and Services Administration (HRSA)	—	113	661	1,416	1,599	1,815	1,917	2,025
Agency for Healthcare Research and Quality	—	8	9	2	2	3	3	2
Office of the Secretary[c]	—	10	6	12	13	15	14	18
Indian Health Service	—	3	4	4	4	4	4	4
Emergency Fund	...	...	...	50	50	50	50	50
Global AIDS Trust Fund	...	...	...	...	...	...	125	99
The International Mother and Child HIV Prevention Initiative[d]	...	...	...	...	...	...	...	40
Centers for Medicare & Medicaid Services	75	780	2,500	4,400	5,000	5,600	6,250	7,150
Social Security Administration[e]	17	...	...	...	...	...	...	...
Ricky Ray Hemophilia Relief Fund (HRSA)[f]	...	...	...	...	75	580	...	...
Social Security Administration[e]	...	239	881	1,158	1,240	1,259	1,351	1,395
Department of Veterans Affairs	8	220	317	401	345	405	391	396
Department of Defense	—	124	110	86	97	108	96	78
Agency for International Development	—	71	120	139	200	430	510	873
Department of Housing and Urban Development	—	—	171	225	232	257	277	292
Office of Personnel Management	—	37	212	266	279	292	297	321
Other departments	—	7	8	10	11	27	27	30
Activity								
Research	75	1,013	1,460	1,900	2,125	2,368	2,614	2,821
Department of Health and Human Services discretionary spending[b]	75	974	1,417	1,869	2,085	2,328	2,580	2,800
Department of Veterans Affairs	—	6	5	7	7	7	8	8
Department of Defense	—	33	38	24	33	33	26	13
Education and prevention	33	591	770	902	998	1,396	1,629	1,940
Department of Health and Human Services discretionary spending[b]	33	460	604	719	751	950	1,091	1,130
Department of Veterans Affairs	—	29	31	30	33	35	35	35
Department of Defense	—	28	12	10	10	17	17	11
Agency for International Development	—	71	120	139	200	380	473	749
Other	—	3	3	4	4	14	13	15
Medical care	83	1,227	3,738	6,595	7,356	8,324	9,117	10,229
Centers for Medicare & Medicaid Services:								
Medicaid (federal share)	70	670	1,500	2,900	3,300	3,700	4,200	4,800
Medicare	5	110	1,000	1,500	1,700	1,900	2,050	2,350
Department of Health and Human Services discretionary spending[b]	—	158	680	1,507	1,711	1,948	2,118	2,212
Department of Veterans Affairs	8	185	281	364	305	363	348	353
Department of Defense	—	63	60	52	54	58	53	54
Agency for International Development	—	—	—	—	—	50	38	124
Office of Personnel Management	—	37	212	266	279	292	297	321
Other	—	4	5	6	7	13	14	15

does not apply to any EMA named and funded before fiscal year 1997.) In fiscal year (FY) 1991, the first year Title I grants were available, there were only nineteen EMAs. In FY 2004 there were fifty-one EMAs in twenty-two states, the District of Columbia, and Puerto Rico. More than $4.8 billion in Title I funding has been allotted from FY 1991 through 2003. In FY 2004 EMAs received $595.3 million. New York ($122.1 million), Los Angeles ($36.6 million), Washington, D.C. ($30 million), and San Francisco ($29.8 million) received the largest grants. (See Table 6.4.)

In fiscal year 2005, the total amount of the Title I awards declined to $587.4 million. The proportionate amounts awarded to some of the EMAs has also declined. New York is slated to receive $117.9 million, San Francisco $28.3 million, and Washington $29.4 million. However, the amount received by Los Angeles has increased to $36.8 million. (See Table 6.4.)

Title II funds are provided to state governments. Ninety percent of Title II funds are distributed on the basis of AIDS patient counts, while 10% are distributed

TABLE 6.3

Federal spending for HIV-related activities, according to agency and type of activity, selected years 1985–2003 [CONTINUED]

[Data are compiled from federal government appropriations]

Agency and type of activity	1985	1990	1995	1999	2000	2001	2002ª	2003
Cash assistance	17	239	1,052	1,383	1,547	2,096	1,628	1,687
Social Security Administration:								
Disability Insurance	12	184	631	828	870	919	961	985
Supplemental Security Income	5	55	250	330	370	340	390	410
Department of Housing and Urban Development	—	—	171	225	232	257	277	292
Ricky Ray Hemophilia Relief Fundᶠ	...	...	...	...	75	580	...	...

—Quantity zero.
. . . Category not applicable.
ªPreliminary figures.
ᵇDiscretionary spending is contrasted with entitlement spending. Medicare and Medicaid are examples of entitlement spending.
ᶜThe Office of the Assistant Secretary for Health prior to fiscal year 1996.
ᵈThe International Mother and Child HIV Prevention Initiative was introduced in 2002 with funding starting in fiscal year 2003.
ᵉPrior to 1995 the Social Security Administration was part of the Department of Health and Human Services.
ᶠThe Ricky Ray Hemophilia Relief Fund was established by the U.S. Congress in 1998 to make compassionate payments to certain individuals who were treated with antihemophilic factor between July 1, 1982 and December 31, 1987, and who contracted HIV. Some family members may also be covered by the fund.

SOURCE: "Table 128. Federal Spending for Human Immunodeficiency Virus (HIV)–Related Activities, According to Agency and Type of Activity, Selected Fiscal Years 1985–2003," in *Health, United States, 2004 with Chartbook on Trends in the Health of Americans*, Centers for Disease Control and Prevention, 2004, http://www.cdc.gov/hiv/stats/2003SurveillanceReport.pdf (accessed July 18, 2005)

through competitive grants awarded to public and nonprofit agencies. More than $6.7 billion in Title II funding was allotted from FY 1991 through 2003. (States that have more than 1% of all AIDS cases reported nationally during the preceding two years must match the federal grant with their own resources. The amount is based on an annual formula.) The totals increased from $845.7 million in FY 2001 to $1.03 billion in 2004. (See Table 6.5.) The states use their Title II funds to contract with service providers for ambulatory (outpatient) health care, insurance coverage, residential and in-home hospice care, transportation to and from appointments, food banks, and home-delivered meals.

In addition to the base award granted under Title II, states receive funds to support AIDS Drug Assistance Programs (ADAPs). ADAPs provide medication to low-income HIV-positive people who are either uninsured or underinsured. (The states may elect to use their Title II funds for their ADAPs.) Beginning in 1996, extra funds were made available for the ADAPs. In FY 1999 a total of $709.9 million (including $461 million for ADAP funding) was allocated for improved health care and support services for people living with HIV/AIDS. Additionally, 1999 was the first year that Guam and the U.S. Virgin Islands received ADAP funding. For FY 2001 the amount earmarked for ADAP was $589 million. FY 2001 also was the first year that 3% of the ADAP allocation was directed to fund supplemental drug grants to states demonstrating severe need.

Title III of the CARE Act funds grants to provide early intervention services and outpatient treatment for low-income, medically underserved people and supports development of quality HIV primary care programs. During 2002 Title III grants served 150,000 patients; 70% were people of color and 30% were women. In fiscal year 2005 the Title III funding will total $25.7 million. Title IV funds link primary health care and social services for women, infants, and children to HIV research and clinical drug trials. For FY 2002, $193.9 million was allocated to Title III programs and $70.9 million for Title IV programs.

As of August 2005, the CARE Act was facing funding reallocation. The U.S. Department of Health and Human Services proposed reauthorizing the act, which would reduce funding to metropolitan areas that have pioneered AIDS treatment efforts and redirect money to states that have been less timely in their response to HIV/AIDS. If approved, the reauthorization would reduce funding in AIDS-intensive states, including New York and California.

Private Insurance and Medicaid

The financing of HIV/AIDS care is increasingly becoming the responsibility of Medicaid, a government program designed to provide medical care for people who fit the criteria for funding. Greater reliance on Medicaid funding is due in large part to the increase in the number of HIV/AIDS cases among intravenous drug users and poor people who are unlikely to be covered by private health insurance. In addition, many patients who once had private insurance through their workplace lost their coverage when the illness made them too sick to work, forcing them to turn to Medicaid and other public programs.

Added to this list are those whose employment or economic status would normally ensure them insurance coverage, but who became virtually ineligible for private health insurance coverage once they tested positive for HIV. Others need assistance because some insurance companies consider HIV infection a "preexisting

TABLE 6.4

Ryan White CARE Act Title I grant awards, 2000–05

Eligible metropolitan area	FY 2000	FY 2001	FY 2002	FY 2003	FY 2004	FY 2005
Atlanta GA	$15,507,832	$15,992,692	$17,554,590	$18,751,178	$18,339,732	$19,126,568
Austin TX	3,575,995	3,922,582	3,946,480	3,995,912	3,800,520	3,851,321
Baltimore MD	15,351,112	16,698,367	17,986,832	21,458,791	19,710,879	19,179,964
Bergen-Passaic NJ	4,626,995	5,234,104	5,313,602	5,203,065	4,814,704	4,376,432
Boston MA	12,469,255	15,363,160	15,198,508	15,398,403	14,848,697	13,651,229
Caguas PR	1,713,686	1,750,404	1,768,847	1,623,395	1,816,647	1,816,497
Chicago IL	19,003,954	22,963,079	23,005,863	23,225,285	25,426,760	24,992,277
Cleveland-Lorain-Elyria OH	3,107,796	3,384,855	3,535,615	3,593,703	3,486,936	3,464,211
Dallas TX	11,077,000	12,098,406	12,001,240	13,205,009	12,820,583	13,038,882
Denver CO	4,581,734	4,840,128	4,741,353	5,035,812	4,529,097	4,305,958
Detroit MI	7,234,813	7,612,631	8,363,876	8,766,530	8,590,281	8,605,663
Dutchess Co. NY	1,208,858	1,362,331	1,271,442	1,337,041	1,231,242	1,222,865
Ft. Lauderdale FL	11,437,539	13,816,037	14,872,845	14,695,524	14,749,550	14,611,634
Ft Worth-Arlington TX	2,968,606	3,298,024	3,376,074	3,503,726	3,373,450	3,502,064
Hartford CT	4,417,574	4,868,180	4,648,410	4,679,151	4,552,237	4,498,360
Houston TX	17,665,434	19,283,756	19,720,190	20,526,823	19,128,572	19,911,575
Jacksonville FL	4,175,873	4,799,813	5,019,332	5,166,800	4,863,093	5,025,194
Jersey City NJ	5,541,714	6,167,889	6,278,761	6,426,456	5,884,194	5,644,838
Kansas City MO	3,064,120	3,386,127	3,328,170	3,138,000	3,240,813	2,786,392
Las Vegas NV	3,689,337	4,455,787	4,231,997	4,658,661	4,473,401	4,531,754
Los Angeles CA	34,683,327	35,020,216	37,962,755	39,994,550	36,644,121	36,834,089
Miami FL	23,450,383	25,385,904	27,097,189	27,024,359	25,540,011	24,551,236
Middlesex-Somerset-Hunterdon NJ	2,750,975	2,888,808	2,925,300	2,991,173	2,723,697	2,689,723
Minneapolis-St. Paul MN	2,826,949	3,216,026	3,220,400	3,255,148	3,093,915	3,011,747
Nassau-Suffolk NY	6,118,736	6,532,144	6,242,641	6,470,593	5,951,789	5,805,121
Newark NJ	14,554,092	16,254,538	17,467,481	17,706,875	15,312,104	15,412,565
New Haven CT	6,261,941	6,944,353	6,644,351	7,545,500	7,069,348	7,050,669
New Orleans LA	5,935,834	6,942,652	7,066,837	7,326,105	6,787,028	7,323,546
New York NY	107,560,148	119,256,891	117,739,488	103,875,412	122,103,117	117,906,710
Norfolk VA	4,089,698	4,736,759	4,906,134	5,168,622	4,820,201	4,726,063
Oakland CA	6,704,657	6,776,406	6,987,208	7,024,473	6,611,607	6,092,561
Orange County CA	4,670,880	4,956,671	5,564,004	5,683,092	5,233,329	5,041,476
Orlando FL	6,007,600	6,497,014	7,225,978	7,329,133	7,821,786	7,963,150
Philadelphia PA	18,134,011	22,114,655	23,522,981	24,744,302	24,448,485	24,051,724
Phoenix AZ	5,001,568	6,575,645	6,422,556	6,867,905	6,814,427	6,467,107
Ponce PR	2,460,695	2,607,961	2,858,721	2,611,677	2,718,331	2,431,319
Portland OR	3,216,312	3,513,044	3,649,120	3,687,601	3,567,475	3,445,252
Riverside-San Bernardino CA	6,913,948	6,940,381	7,428,435	7,199,843	6,823,183	6,362,841
Sacramento CA	2,744,171	2,899,765	2,840,714	2,660,029	2,968,051	2,782,514
St. Louis MO	4,239,080	4,432,316	4,767,604	5,068,856	4,371,154	4,494,789
San Antonio TX	3,163,374	3,862,398	3,876,586	3,806,139	3,833,443	3,893,845
San Diego CA	9,071,625	10,577,352	10,436,496	10,765,303	10,287,797	9,741,708
San Francisco CA	35,246,477	35,771,651	33,561,470	33,941,235	29,849,780	28,297,777
San Jose CA	2,612,060	2,866,655	2,754,005	2,798,524	2,656,550	2,497,465
San Juan PR	13,558,330	15,094,482	16,235,174	14,772,898	14,732,565	14,695,304
Santa Rosa-Petaluma CA	1,152,406	1,206,194	1,131,226	1,106,742	1,107,428	1,049,715
Seattle WA	5,488,688	5,852,286	5,978,779	6,286,678	5,842,615	5,631,611
Tampa-St. Petersburg FL	8,016,131	8,595,830	8,530,778	8,856,949	8,719,669	9,196,277
Vineland-Millville-Bridgeton NJ	684,897	807,157	910,779	810,259	847,898	875,354
Washington DC	19,903,750	24,507,346	25,980,259	27,871,807	26,951,014	29,431,967
West Palm Beach FL	7,169,030	7,795,848	9,156,524	9,871,953	9,408,695	9,526,597
Totals	**$526,811,000**	**$582,727,700**	**$597,256,000**	**$599,513,000**	**$595,342,001**	**$587,425,500**

SOURCE: Adapted from "HHS Awards $595 Million for AIDS Cure in Major Urban Areas," U.S. Department of Health and Human Services, March 4, 2004, http://www.hhs.gov/news/press/2004pres/20040301a.html (accessed July 18, 2005); "HHS Awards More Than $1 Billion to States to Help Provide Care, Services and Prescription Drugs for People with HIV/AIDS," U.S. Department of Health and Human Services, April 1, 2004, http://www.hhs.gov/news/press/2004pres/20040401b.html (accessed July 18, 2005)

condition," making it ineligible for payment of claims. Even insurance companies that do cover HIV treatment often impose caps, limiting coverage to relatively small dollar amounts.

The HIV/AIDS epidemic has prompted private insurers to add an HIV antibody screening test for people who are not joining insurance programs through groups or employers. These "individual enrollees"—who make up 15% of all people in the insurance market—are required to take medical exams to prove they are "insurable." In the early 1990s California, Massachusetts, and the District of Columbia initially banned the use of HIV antibody testing for private insurance purposes but reversed the ban in the storm of resulting controversy.

Death Benefits

Since 1988 an industry has developed that offers dying AIDS patients the opportunity to collect a portion of their life insurance benefits before they die, either to pay for

TABLE 6.5

Ryan White CARE Act Title II grant awards, 2000–05

State	FY 2000	FY 2001	FY 2002	FY 2003	FY 2004	FY 2005
Alabama	$8,223,550	$9,014,379	$10,132,580	$10,867,008	$11,317,534	$11,881,914
Alaska	644,658	863,456	898,686	926,023	974,705	1,006,313
Arizona	7,876,550	9,111,778	10,130,689	11,255,601	11,648,614	12,732,077
Arkansas	3,729,267	3,970,060	4,397,016	4,933,831	4,933,831	5,161,119
California	106,594,028	108,836,753	115,580,982	118,274,998	121,425,527	121,734,064
Colorado	6,501,977	6,637,149	7,239,683	7,447,255	7,759,634	7,759,634
Connecticut	12,473,062	13,071,734	13,873,014	14,915,598	15,175,723	15,746,598
Delaware	3,444,082	3,714,668	4,549,172	5,129,211	5,340,795	5,432,326
Dist. of Columbia	12,208,813	13,851,117	15,492,398	16,875,124	18,323,488	18,951,519
Florida	84,151,932	90,174,364	99,913,339	108,800,440	111,668,948	116,883,905
Georgia	24,609,445	26,149,782	28,689,786	32,523,811	33,354,271	36,312,311
Hawaii	2,714,578	2,832,895	2,879,231	3,134,711	3,298,130	3,298,130
Idaho	637,862	883,461	914,852	940,179	964,689	965,496
Illinois	23,741,440	26,962,344	29,041,633	32,061,756	34,870,568	36,007,864
Indiana	7,813,244	8,150,351	9,607,370	10,080,837	11,402,950	11,631,445
Iowa	1,597,254	1,684,688	1,886,371	2,046,335	2,067,375	2,111,150
Kansas	2,680,639	2,856,155	2,993,080	3,061,160	3,061,160	3,130,712
Kentucky	4,679,465	5,048,838	5,877,450	6,566,479	6,688,723	6,962,984
Louisiana	14,659,595	15,606,237	17,803,081	19,165,624	21,324,721	23,096,176
Maine	1,053,098	1,165,524	1,222,848	1,291,963	1,333,909	1,333,909
Maryland	23,625,388	25,567,961	28,539,346	33,236,307	34,509,971	36,055,252
Massachusetts	15,135,145	17,667,413	19,027,859	20,165,312	20,190,874	20,190,874
Michigan	11,836,551	12,389,033	13,817,447	14,902,329	15,455,849	15,983,050
Minnesota	3,429,038	3,583,168	3,930,918	4,041,505	4,059,707	4,183,467
Mississippi	5,940,732	6,824,201	7,994,828	8,927,096	9,454,950	10,514,013
Missouri	8,842,764	9,100,570	10,041,335	10,231,106	10,250,137	10,500,632
Montana	493,995	766,328	784,249	798,932	810,671	810,671
Nebraska	1,363,635	1,419,699	1,610,116	1,735,366	1,757,215	1,757,215
Nevada	4,962,828	5,341,517	5,768,265	6,248,392	6,456,309	6,654,115
New Hampshire	927,722	1,137,986	1,170,914	1,225,589	1,257,028	1,281,115
New Jersey	40,762,441	42,500,140	45,652,579	47,117,129	47,641,537	47,641,537
New Mexico	2,684,197	2,842,890	3,042,298	3,338,463	3,338,463	3,489,677
New York	138,462,204	146,425,361	153,793,751	166,416,534	169,263,213	171,786,592
North Carolina	13,337,097	14,419,871	16,541,998	18,905,269	21,144,376	21,945,256
North Dakota	183,474	287,207	288,717	292,543	292,543	306,199
Ohio	12,862,596	13,458,225	14,653,307	15,732,171	16,762,266	16,794,093
Oklahoma	4,285,048	4,506,022	5,426,183	5,923,857	5,923,857	5,928,122
Oregon	4,722,939	4,836,281	5,266,094	5,719,559	5,902,627	5,943,054
Pennsylvania	26,896,745	29,152,465	32,266,464	37,124,991	38,316,474	39,891,047
Rhode Island	2,574,101	2,637,933	2,981,815	3,104,681	3,189,276	3,189,276
South Carolina	13,250,895	14,671,072	16,671,207	18,549,396	19,323,103	20,521,015
South Dakota	233,352	338,771	372,293	391,032	705,706	727,255
Tennessee	11,468,392	12,886,043	16,464,366	21,178,234	21,178,234	21,178,234
Texas	56,932,045	59,601,232	63,832,668	68,629,133	70,065,527	73,889,574
Utah	2,426,761	2,623,772	3,111,672	3,235,191	3,235,191	3,235,191
Vermont	510,156	787,721	838,895	883,059	883,059	883,059
Virginia	14,845,195	16,293,263	18,955,891	20,375,565	20,817,878	21,086,328
Washington	9,019,810	9,311,929	10,243,929	10,986,852	11,121,586	11,198,763
West Virginia	1,462,626	1,550,249	1,702,361	1,943,767	2,021,847	2,095,875
Wisconsin	4,242,502	4,338,571	4,874,441	5,183,308	5,214,471	5,227,607
Wyoming	205,536	329,954	340,041	350,383	360,347	369,918
Guam	38,809	116,169	118,503	132,268	135,839	142,852
Puerto Rico	25,647,632	26,646,201	28,814,408	30,748,881	31,098,002	31,098,002
Virgin Islands	667,110	759,549	772,935	976,601	976,601	976,602
Total grants	**$794,314,000**	**$845,704,500**	**$923,088,000**	**$999,308,000**	**$1,030,309,284**	**$1,059,874,618**

Note: 2002 and 2003 totals include grants made in U.S. Pacific territories besides Guam.

SOURCE: Adapted from "HHS Awards More Than $1 Billion to States to Help Provide Care, Services and Prescription Drugs for People with HIV/AIDS," U.S. Department of Health and Human Services, April 1, 2004, http://www.hhs.gov/news/press/2004pres/20040401b.html (accessed July 18, 2005); "HHS Awards Almost $1.7 Billion for HIV/AIDS Cure," U.S. Department of Health and Human Services, March 2, 2005, http://www.hhs.gov/news/press/2005pres/20050302.html (accessed July 18, 2005)

their treatment or to spend as they wish during their remaining time. These viatical (money for necessities given to a person dying or in danger of death) settlements are reached when an insured person sells his or her life insurance policy to an independent insurance company at a reduced or discounted price. This enables the patient to have some cash from the policy while he or she is still alive. After the patient dies, the company that bought the policy is paid the full death benefits. Regulators with the Securities and Exchange Commission are scrutinizing some practices that they say may victimize AIDS patients.

Some larger companies such as Prudential offer policy holders more than 90% of their policy payouts, but only with a physician's certification that they have less than six months to live. Smaller companies usually pay 50 to 80% of the benefit payable at death, although they will pay benefits to people who still have up to five years to live. The longer the person is expected to live, the less the cash disbursement they receive.

Most insurers will not write new life insurance policies for people known to have AIDS. But the insurance industry had paid out more than $640 million in death benefits by 2002 on policies of already-insured people who died of AIDS. At least one company does offer life insurance policies to some people infected with HIV, provided they meet certain eligibility requirements.

TREATMENT RESEARCH

Medical and pharmaceutical research to develop and conduct clinical trials of antiretroviral drugs is expensive. In 2002 the National Institutes of Health (NIH) spent an estimated $2.7 billion on AIDS research, while it spent approximately $630 million to investigate breast cancer and $263 million for research on strokes.

Decisions about how much is spent to research a particular disease are not based solely on how many people develop the disease or die from it. Rightly or wrongly, economists base the societal value of an individual on his or her earning potential and productivity—the ability to contribute to society as a worker. The bulk of the people who die from heart disease, stroke, and cancer are older adults. Many have retired from the workforce and their potential economic productivity is often minimal. This economic measure of present and future financial productivity should not be misinterpreted as a "casting-off" of older adults; instead, it is simply an economic measure of present and future financial productivity.

In contrast, AIDS patients are usually much younger and die in their twenties, thirties, and forties. Until they develop AIDS the potential productivity of these people, measured in economic terms, is high. The number of work years lost when they die is considerable. Using this economic equation to determine how disease research should be funded, it may be considered economically wise to invest more money to research AIDS since the losses, measured in potential work years rather than lives, are so much greater.

The primary goals of HIV/AIDS therapy are to prolong life and improve its quality. While in the early days of AIDS research a cure for the disease was envisioned, few researchers by the early 2000s realistically expected any drug to cure HIV infection. The bottom-line objective became making the virus less deadly by foiling its efforts to reproduce within the body.

A major obstacle to the discovery of such treatments is the cost of drug research and development. Pharmaceutical manufacturers spend millions of dollars researching and developing new medicines. According to the Pharmaceutical Research and Manufacturers of America, since 1992 U.S. pharmaceutical companies have consistently spent more money each year on research and development (R&D) activities than the annual budget of the National Institutes of Health. For example, in 2002 the estimated pharmaceutical R&D budget was $32 billion, while the entire NIH budget (research and other activities) was $24 billion. Furthermore, private-sector spending has been growing faster than government spending since 1995.

As of 2005, pharmaceutical companies were testing seventy-nine medications for HIV/AIDS and associated conditions. The successful candidates will complement the eighty-two medications that were approved since the 1980s.

A pharmaceutical manufacturer must cover the cost not only of R&D for the approximately three out of ten drugs that succeed, but also for many of the drugs—seven out of ten—that fail to make it to the marketplace. Because of this cost, once a new drug receives U.S. Food and Drug Administration (FDA) approval, its manufacturer ordinarily holds a patent or gains exclusivity rights, which guarantee it will be the sole marketer for a specified time (usually from three to twenty years) in order to recoup its investment. During this time, the drug is priced much higher than if other manufacturers were allowed to compete by producing generic versions of the same drug. In contrast to the original manufacturer, the generic manufacturer does not have to pay for the successes and failures that occurred in the drug development pathway or pursue the complicated, time-consuming process of seeking FDA approval. The producer of generic drugs has the formula and must simply manufacture the drugs properly. Because of the lower cost of the generic drug after the original patent or exclusivity period has expired, competition among pharmaceutical manufacturers generally lowers the price. HIV/AIDS drugs are granted seven years of exclusivity under legislation aimed at encouraging research and promoting development of new treatments.

The issue of patent protection for HIV/AIDS drugs is understandably contentious. Pharmaceutical manufacturers and others argue that patent protection is necessary to allow for the financial investments necessary to breed innovation. However, to those directly affected by HIV/AIDS, and those governments or health care systems that provide care, the enormous costs can be infuriating, especially with the knowledge that generic drugs carrying a lower price tag are possible. In the developing world, the need for less expensive HIV/AIDS drugs is urgent.

Indeed, reflecting this urgency, a November 2002 meeting of the World Trade Organization (WTO) adopted a resolution affirming the right of WTO member countries to do whatever they deem necessary to protect public health, including overriding pharmaceutical patents. In May 2003 the government of Zimbabwe declared a national emergency for six months over the HIV/AIDS pandemic, enabling it to purchase and make available generic versions of HIV/AIDS drugs that are still under patent protection. Prior to this, the passage of the Kenya Industrial Property Bill 2001 allowed the importation and production of more affordable medicines for HIV/AIDS in that country.

FDA-APPROVED DRUGS

The first drug thought to delay symptoms was zidovudine (ZDV; formerly known as azidothymidine, or AZT). While initially promising, ZDV's effects were found to be temporary at best. Several other drugs work on the same principle as ZDV—exclusion of HIV from the host chromosome. A new class of drugs called protease inhibitors (PIs) appears to keep HIV already in the host cells from reproducing. PIs block the ability of HIV to mature and infect new cells by suppressing a protein enzyme of the virus, called protease, which is crucial to the progression of HIV. One study conducted by Merck shows that a combination of Crixivan and two other AIDS drugs reduces virus load by more than 99% in patients with T cell counts between 50 and 400 virus particles per cubic millimeter.

Even if the effectiveness of PIs proves to be transient, they should improve patients' prospects simply by creating more roadblocks for HIV, which mutates so rapidly that it becomes resistant to most drugs when the drugs are used alone. Even if a cure is never found, new and better drugs used in various combinations may make HIV infection a chronic but manageable disease, much like diabetes.

The cost, however, is high. PIs range from about $4,800 to $8,000 for a year's supply. When combined with ZDV or any of the other commonly used antiretroviral drugs, such as lamivudine (3TC), zalcitabine (ddC), didanosine (ddI), or stavudine (d4T), the cost is approximately $18,000 per year. Government programs and private insurers alike are looking for ways to pay for, and in some cases avoid paying for, these new therapies. As Moises Agosto of the National Minority AIDS Council in Washington, D.C., notes, though the drugs may be approved, people may still not be able to use the new treatments if programs cannot afford them.

Types of Antiretroviral Agents

As of 2005 the FDA accepted the following classes of antiretroviral agents for treatment of HIV/AIDS.

PROTEASE INHIBITORS. The following are PIs:

- Indinavir, manufactured by Merck and sold under the brand name Crixivan

- Ritonavir, manufactured by Abbott Laboratories and sold under the brand name Norvir

- Saquinavir, manufactured by Roche Pharmaceuticals and sold under the brand names Invirase and Fortovase

- Nelfinavir, manufactured by Agouron Pharmaceuticals and sold under the brand name Viracept

- Amprenavir, manufactured by GlaxoSmithKline and sold under the brand name Agenerase

- Atazanavir, manufactured by Bristol-Myers Squibb and sold under the brand name Reyataz

- Fosamprenavir calcium, manufactured by GlaxoSmithKline and Vertex Pharmaceuticals and sold under the brand name Lexiva

Drugs formulated with combinations of two or more protease inhibitors also have received FDA approval:

- Lopinavir and ritonavir, manufactured by Abbott Laboratories and sold under the brand name Kaletra; for use in adult and pediatric patients

- Abacavir, retrovir, and lamivudine in a fixed dose combination, manufactured by GlaxoSmithKline and sold under the brand name Trizivir

NUCLEOSIDE ANALOGS. Nucleoside analogs (NAs) were among the first compounds shown to be effective against viral infections. Research in the 1970s led to the development of the drug acyclovir, which is still being used to treat herpes infections. The first four anti-HIV drugs to be approved—ZDV (at one time called AZT), didanosine, dideoxycytosine, and stavudine—were NAs.

As their name implies, NAs exert their action based on their three-dimensional structure, which mimics the structure of the nucleoside building blocks of DNA. By becoming incorporated into DNA as the molecule is replicated, the analogs can preserve the structure of DNA but make it impossible for the HIV to use its reverse transcriptase to hijack the host replication machinery to make new viral copies.

As of 2005, the following NAs have received FDA approval for use with HIV/AIDS:

- ZDV, manufactured by GlaxoSmithKline and sold under the brand name Retrovir

- Didanosine (also called dideoxyinosine, or ddI), manufactured by Bristol-Myers Squibb and sold under the brand name Videx

- Zalcitabine (also called dideoxycytosine, or ddC), manufactured by Roche Pharmaceuticals and sold under the brand name Hivid

- Stavudine (D4T), manufactured by Bristol-Myers Squibb and sold under the brand name Zerit

- Lamivudine (3TC), manufactured by GlaxoSmithKline and sold under the brand name Epivir

- Abacavir succinate, manufactured by GlaxoSmithKline and sold under the brand name Ziagen

- A combination of lamivudine and abacavir, manufactured by GlaxoSmithKline and sold under the brand name Epizicom

- A combination of emtricitabine and tenofovir disoproxil fumarate, manufactured by Gilead Sciences and sold under the brand name Truvada

NONNUCLEOSIDE REVERSE TRANSCRIPTASE INHIBITORS. Another class of antiretroviral drugs approved in the late 1990s is nonnucleoside reverse transcriptase inhibitors (NNRTIs). NNRTI compounds slow down the process of the reverse transcriptase enzyme that allows the virus to become part of the infected cell's nucleus. The compounds accomplish this by binding to the viral enzyme, which blocks the ability of the enzyme to function. As of 2005 there were three NNRTIs approved for use by the FDA:

- Nevirapine, manufactured by Boehringer Ingelheim and sold under the brand name Viramune

- Delavirdine, manufactured by Pfizer and sold under the brand name Rescriptor

- Efavirenz, manufactured by Bristol-Myers Squibb and sold under the brand name Sustiva

- Amprenavir, manufactured by GlaxoSmithKline and sold under the brand name Combivir

- Emtricitabine, manufactured by Gilead Sciences and sold under the brand name Emtriva

NUCLEOTIDE ANALOGS. Like nucleoside analogs, nucleotide analogs also inhibit the HIV reverse transcriptase. However, the molecular mechanism of this inhibition is different from nucleoside analogs. Specifically, nucleotide analogs are active without modification, while the nucleoside inhibitors only work in cells that have the machinery to add a phosphorus group to the compounds. This may allow nucleotide analogs to be active in a wider range of HIV-infected cells than nucleoside inhibitors. Nucleotide analogs have the advantages of only needing to be taken once a day and show some effectiveness against resistant HIV. However, serious side effects such as kidney damage and eye inflammation have been reported with some nucleotide analogs.

In October 2001 the FDA approved Viread (tenofovir disoproxil fumarate) as the first and, as of 2005, only nucleotide analog for HIV treatment. Intended for use in combination with other antiretroviral drugs, the new drug has been shown to reduce HIV replication. But there are not yet long-term study results to demonstrate whether Viread effectively inhibits the clinical progression of HIV.

AN ANTI-FUSION DRUG. As of 2005, one drug that interferes with the fusion of HIV with the host cell membrane has been approved by the FDA. Enfuvitide, which is manufactured by Roche and Trimeris, is sold under the brand name Fuzeon.

Aggressive Treatment

With new drugs in the anti-HIV/AIDS arsenal, many people with HIV/AIDS who had given up hope of effective treatment returned to clinics and doctors' offices. While treatment guidelines previously promoted early intervention with ZDV, recommended treatment now combines PIs with other antiretroviral drugs. Treatment recommendations change rapidly in response to the development of new drugs and clinical trials indicating the effectiveness of different combinations of antiretroviral drugs. Researchers are acting quickly to develop new mixtures of the recently approved and older drugs. Because HIV mutates to resist any drug it faces, including all PIs, researchers find that varying the combination of drugs prescribed can "fool" the virus before it has time to mutate.

Another approach to treatment, presented in an article published in the February 15, 2000, issue of the *Annals of Internal Medicine* by Keith Henry, suggests that overly aggressive antiretroviral therapy in the early stages of the disease may expose patients to unpleasant side effects and cause their systems to build resistance. Henry recommends a more cautious strategy: a long-term, patient-focused approach that includes delaying initial therapy, planned interruptions in drug dose administration, therapy switching, and immune-based therapy. In October 2003 the European Medicines Agency advised doctors not to start HIV patients on the aggressive didanosine–lamivudine–tenovir triple-drug combination, since no compelling improvement had been noted in those receiving the treatment.

Patients undergoing therapy with new drugs or drug combinations must be highly disciplined. For instance, Crixivan must be taken on an empty stomach, every eight hours, not less than two hours before or after a meal, and with large amounts of water to prevent development of kidney stones. Patients must also be careful to never skip doses of Crixivan, otherwise HIV will quickly grow immune to its effect. (Crixivan has been found to generate cross-resistance, meaning it made patients resistant to other PIs.) Invirase must be taken in large doses. Norvir must be carefully prescribed and administered because it interacts negatively with some antifungals and antibiotics used by AIDS patients. Because there are numerous minor and serious risks associated with use of these drugs, patients must be closely monitored.

The difficulty of dealing with a complicated regimen of daily medication and maintaining the personal resolve to continue the regimen are issues for HIV/AIDS patients. Henry argues that more support should be given to those health care professionals (such as nurses and pharmacists) who educate patients and assist them in maintaining their complicated daily medication schedules. During 2000 many combined HIV/AIDS medication regimens could be administered two to three times per day, and once-a-day regimens may be possible in the near future. Such a possibility, according to the researchers, may lead to improved adherence to treatment and quality of life for people with HIV/AIDS.

Lingering Questions

As observed earlier, the success of PIs may prove transient. Studies conducted by drug companies that produce the PIs show that viral loads decrease to undetectable levels for at least a few months whether the patients have been HIV-positive for a few weeks or a few years. Because the drugs were allowed to be used under the FDA's accelerated approval program—a fast-track approval after safety and efficacy are demonstrated in a single clinical trial—some investigators question their long-term efficacy. If each PI is able to suppress HIV for only a little while, critics ask, then are HIV/AIDS patients any better off?

Other questions persist. Even though HIV patients treated with PIs may have no detectable HIV in their blood, might it still be present in their tissue? Will drug-resistant strains of the virus emerge over time? Will these powerful drugs cause harmful side effects if taken for long periods? Is it safe to switch from one drug to another once there is resistance? Studies are underway and more are planned to determine the optimal therapy and when it should begin.

AIDS and Marijuana

Marijuana (*Cannabis sativa*) is an herb that has become infamous for the "high" it can cause, due to a constituent chemical called tetrahydrocannabinal (THC). Until the late 1930s the beneficial properties of marijuana to relieve pain and increase appetite were recognized, and the drug was used medically in the United States. By the 1970s, however, marijuana's medical benefits were considered to be far outweighed by the potential for abuse, and laws banning its use were enacted in the United States and other countries.

As recently as June 2005, the U.S. Supreme Court ruled that the medical use of marijuana is illegal under federal law. However, some states have passed laws that permit the use of the drug for medically approved reasons, such as relief for pain and nausea. In Canada marijuana use for cancer and AIDS patients is legal; in fact, the patients obtain the drug from federal government-grown plants.

In 1992 the FDA approved a version of marijuana for medical use. The product, called Marinol, contains synthetic THC and is available by prescription. Administration of THC in a pill form allows patients to avoid the inhalation of marijuana smoke, which can contain many potentially noxious chemicals. Many AIDS patients, however, claim that Marinol is too weak to alleviate their symptoms.

Marijuana's ability to stimulate appetite and suppress nausea have made it an attractive adjunct to HIV/AIDS therapy. Nonetheless, opposition to the medical use of the drug still exists. This is particularly true of the proposal to make the traditional cigarette (or reefer) form of marijuana available for medical use. In August 2005 the U.S. Drug Enforcement Administration heard presentations from advocates and critics of a proposal to allow the FDA to decide if marijuana should be reclassified as a prescription drug.

THE DISCOVERY OF AN HIV-RESISTANT GENE

In August 1996 scientists working independently at the Aaron Diamond AIDS Research Center in New York City and the Free University of Brussels, Belgium, announced that some white people have genes that may protect them from HIV no matter how many times they are exposed to the virus. The researchers hope the findings could lead to new HIV/AIDS therapies or to the development of pills or injections to prevent HIV.

The researchers discovered that a gene called CCR5 is associated with HIV resistance. The gene codes for a protein called CC chemokine receptor 5 (CCR5) that is located on the surface of host cells including macrophages, monocytes, and T cells. HIV exploits this protein by using it as a receptor to bind to, and subsequently infect, cells such as T cells. The CCR5 mutation blocks the manufacture of CCR5. Thus, HIV loses its surface target and cannot invade the immune system.

Subsequent studies conducted in the United States found that one in one hundred people inherits two copies of this gene—one from each parent—and is completely immune to HIV infection. One in five people with only one copy of the CCR5 gene can become infected, but remains healthy two to three years longer than those without the altered gene. This may be because he or she has half as many CCR5 receptors as is normal, which limits or slows the spread of the virus.

Research studies in the United States have found that the gene is most common in white Americans (10 to 15% of the population). It is rarely found in black Americans and almost never in Africans or Asians, perhaps reflecting the origins of the mutation.

Certain populations appear to be resistant to HIV because they lack or have a mutated form of the CCR5 receptor. Most populations that carry the mutant CCR5 gene come from Europe, and there are indications that the mutation arose only about seven hundred years ago. For a mutation to be sustained in a population at a rate of 10%, there must be some benefit bestowed by the mutation. It is likely nothing to do with HIV, since HIV did not appear until the middle of the twentieth century.

Exactly what the selective pressure was that caused the appearance of the CCR5 mutation is debatable. A prevailing theory has been that the selective pressure was the bubonic plague. But new research leads to the proposal that smallpox was the trigger. Which of these, if either, is true remains to be determined.

Research is also underway to learn more about another gene—CCR2—that, when expressed dominantly, appears to slow the progression of AIDS.

NEW RESEARCH

The Thymus Gland and the Immune System

One of the next major challenges in the fight against HIV/AIDS is reviving a deteriorated immune system. Without a healthy immune system, HIV/AIDS patients will not be able to recover from the disease, even if a cure is found. Researchers theorize that it may be possible to rejuvenate a wasted immune system. The key to this is the thymus gland, which is located next to the heart behind the breastbone. The thymus gland is where T cells mature. When mature, the T cells fight infections in the body. But when HIV invades the body, the virus uses the T cell to replicate itself. The T cell does not survive this process and the whole immune system collapses, leaving the HIV-infected patient susceptible to rare and often deadly opportunistic infections.

Until the late 1990s it was thought that the thymus gland was only active during the first thirty years of life and that no new T cells were made thereafter. In recent years researchers have observed that the new drug combinations, often called "cocktails," seem to be able to boost the number of T cells. No one, however, knows where these new cells are coming from. Currently, doctors use artificial means to increase the number of T cells in HIV-infected persons. If the adult body can

indeed manufacture new T cells, it may be possible to restore the immune system.

Morning-After Treatment

HIV has now been classified as a communicable sexually transmitted disease in the United States. A few doctors are beginning to prescribe some of the drugs used to treat established infections as "morning-after" pills in an attempt to prevent transmission of the virus after risky sexual encounters. As of 2005, there is no scientific consensus on the validity of this approach, and the medications are not licensed for this use. But other forms of HIV are halted by prompt use of the drugs, encouraging some doctors to give it a try. For example, an antiretroviral drug regimen given to hospital personnel following an accidental needle stick from an HIV-infected patient seems to reduce the one in two hundred risk of transmission by about 80%. Similarly, antiretroviral treatment given to HIV-infected pregnant women reduces the risk of transmission to the newborn baby from one in four to less than one in ten.

This "off-label" use of potent PIs in an attempt to prevent the spread of HIV, however, is controversial. All drugs used in the treatment of HIV have side effects, some of which may be potentially life threatening. Furthermore, some researchers fear that if people believe morning-after treatment will prevent HIV infection, they may stop taking precautions, such as using condoms, to prevent exposure to HIV. Others feel that the treatment is not appropriate as a preventive measure for people exposed to ongoing risk, such as relationships where only one partner is infected, because the drugs are too toxic. Other methods, such as the continued use of condoms, would be much safer.

Finally, post-exposure treatment is expensive. The costs of two or three drugs taken for a month, plus laboratory tests and visits to the doctor, may run as high as $1,000. Of course, this is a fraction of the cost for lifetime treatment of HIV infection and certainly money well spent if it prevents a person from acquiring the virus.

Some researchers say the morning-after treatment could save lives. The drugs themselves will save some lives, and the offer of treatment will bring people who are at high risk for acquiring HIV into environments where they can get counseling and care. In San Francisco, California, post-exposure treatment is offered to victims of rape as a matter of course. Some doctors feel that if the treatment does not work to prevent the disease, it may work to at least treat it as early as possible. Though there is disagreement about the effectiveness and wisdom of widespread use of post-exposure treatment, nearly all researchers and health care providers agree that for sexually active people the best prevention is the use of condoms.

Additional Research

There are several promising directions in HIV/AIDS treatment and research. Simplified medication regimens may improve adherence to treatment, and structured treatment interruptions allow the body to recover from the effects of medications. Structured treatment interruptions might, according to the theory, allow the body to regain immunity to HIV during breaks from the medication schedule. Other studies focus on better understanding of HIV-specific immunity and how to retain or restore it, as well as research into nutritional deficiencies that might accelerate the disease among some patients.

IN SEARCH OF A VACCINE

Some pharmaceutical companies claim that the high costs of research and development and the relatively low return on their investments (since the period of patent protection is limited to seven years) leave little financial incentive to develop new HIV/AIDS drugs. And development of such drugs is, for better or worse, an economically driven, rather than strictly humanitarian, enterprise. Similarly, the companies allege that they have little economic motivation to research and develop HIV vaccines. In February 1996 Anthony Fauci, the head of NIAID, released guidelines to promote cooperation between the government and private industry. The plan's goal was to overcome the alleged unfavorable market forces that have caused some companies to abandon research of potential HIV vaccines.

Such vaccine efforts continue. At the beginning of 2003 NIAID and the international HIV Vaccine Trials Network announced an agreement with Merck & Co., a leading manufacturer of anti-HIV compounds, to support the evaluation of promising HIV vaccines. To date, thirty potential vaccines have been evaluated.

In 2005 fifteen vaccine trials involving more than thirty-six hundred participants were in progress, according to the HIV Vaccine Trials Network and the Pharmaceutical Manufacturers of America. (See Table 6.6.) One of the candidate vaccine trials is taking place in the countries of Brazil, Haiti, Peru, and Trinidad and Tobago. Two vaccine trials are underway in South Africa and Botswana. Two other trials are international in scope. Finally, thirteen vaccine trials are ongoing in the United States. While most of the trials are small-scale (phase I) trials, two large-scale phase III trials are underway and two other trials may enter phase III testing.

The design of the vaccines currently under trial is varied. Eight of the vaccines use a weakened and medically safe version of viruses as a delivery vehicle to carry various HIV genes into the human participants. The hope is that antibody production to the HIV critical proteins encoded by these genes will occur, and that this production will offer protection from HIV infection. Six other vaccines use a DNA plasmid to ferry HIV genes into the human participants; the aim again is to stimulate antibody production.

There are problems of experimental design and ethical considerations involved in vaccine trials using human volunteers. Most volunteers for the vaccine have behaviors that put them at risk for contracting HIV. Some may mistakenly believe that participating in the clinical trial of an experimental vaccine—which may be a vaccine or a placebo—protects them and, with a false sense of security, they may resume high-risk behaviors.

If these volunteers contract HIV during the clinical trial, scientists cannot be sure whether it is from risky behaviors or from the experimental vaccine (some vaccines may contain live HIV because a weakened version of the virus itself is used to stimulate the body's immune system to act against the virus). When volunteers contract HIV during trials, the testing is abandoned. On the other hand, volunteers may reduce their risks so successfully that they are never exposed to HIV, leaving the vaccine nothing to fight. This paradox is unique to HIV/AIDS research and frustrates scientists.

Despite optimistic projections in the early 1990s that a vaccine would be found by 1995, a considerable number of promising experimental HIV vaccines have proven ineffective against strains of HIV taken from infected people. Researchers reported developing antibodies that worked successfully against HIV grown in test tubes, but in every case they failed when used against HIV in human beings. NIAID head Anthony Fauci commented that the results of the initial vaccine research were "cause for some sober reflection." As of 2005, none of the candidate vaccines has shown sufficient promise to warrant manufacture, approval, and use.

Nonetheless, Robert Gallo, one of the co-discoverers of HIV and the director of the Institute of Human Virology at the University of Maryland, Baltimore, is cautiously optimistic about the development of the HIV vaccine. Speaking at the first World Congress on Men's Health in Vienna, Austria, in October 2001, Gallo predicted that one of the vaccines then under investigation would likely be successful. Still, those in need will have to wait for this optimism to bear fruit. At that time Gallo said he believed an effective HIV vaccine was "realistically at least five years away."

The First Large-Scale Human Test

In June 1998 the FDA granted permission to VaxGen Inc. of San Francisco to conduct the world's first full-scale test of a vaccine to prevent HIV infection. The VaxGen vaccine—a genetically engineered molecule designated AIDSvax—had been found safe in tests involving twelve hundred volunteers in March 1992, with

TABLE 6.6

Summary of current HIV vaccine trials, 2005

Product name	Sponsor	Indication	Development status
AG-702	Antigenics New York, NY	Genital herpes	Phase I (212) 332-4774
AIDS vaccine	United Biomedical Hauppauge, NY	HIV infection	Phase I (631) 273-2828
AIDS VAX®	VaxGen Brisbane, CA	HIV infection prophylaxis	Phase III (650) 624-1000
ALVAC™ (vCP 1452)	Aventis Pasteur Swiftwater, PA	HIV infection prophylaxis and immunotherapy	Phase II (570) 839-4267
ALVAC™ (vCP 1521)	Aventis Pasteur Swiftwater, PA	HIV infection prophylaxis and immunotherapy	Phase III (570) 839-4267
AVX101 (HIV vaccine)	AlphaVax Rsch. Triangle Park, NC	HIV infection	Phase I (919) 595-0400
EP HIV-1090	Epimmune San Diego, CA	HIV-1 therapy	Phase I (858) 860-2515
Genital herpes vaccine	AuRx Glen Burnie, MD	Treatment of genital herpes	Phase I/II completed (410) 590-7610
HIVA.DNA-MVA	International AIDS Vaccine Initiative New York, NY	HIV-1 prophylaxis	Phase I/II (212) 847-1111
HIV recombinant vaccine	GlaxoSmithKline Philadelphia, PA Rsch. Triangle Park, NC	HIV prophylaxis	Phase I (888) 825-5249
HIV vaccine	Emory Vaccine Center Atlanta, GA GeoVax Atlanta, GA NIAID Bethesda, MD	HIV infection	Phase I
HIV vaccine	Merck Whitehouse Station, NJ	Prevention and treatment of HIV infection/AIDS	Phase I (800) 672-6372
Recombinant vaccine	Therion Biologics Cambridge, MA	AIDS	Phase I (617) 475-7253
Simplirix recombinant vaccine	GlaxoSmithKline Philadelphia, PA Rsch. Triangle Park, NC	Genital herpes prophylaxis	Phase III (888) 825-5249
Tat toxoid	Aventis Pasteur Swiftwater, PA	HIV infection prophylaxis and immunotherapy	Phase I (570) 839-4267

Note: The content of this survey has been obtained through government and industry sources based on the latest information. Survey current as of November 7, 2003. The information may not be comprehensive.

SOURCE: "Vaccines," in *2004 Survey: Medicines in Development for HIV/AIDS*, Pharmaceutical Research and Manufacturers of America, 2003, http://www .phrma.org/newmedicines/resources/2003-11-23.120.pdf (accessed July 18, 2005)

more than 99% of the vaccinated participants producing antibodies. The 1998 test involved five thousand volunteers in forty clinics throughout the United States and Canada, and twenty-five hundred volunteers in sixteen clinics in Thailand.

AIDSvax is made from part of HIV's outer coat, specifically a molecule called gp120. The molecule functions in the attachment of the virus to host cells. The vaccine did not contain the intact virus, only the gp120 protein from two strains of HIV. (Previous vaccines had used one strain.) The two strains of the vaccine that were tested in North America are made with strains common in North America. The vaccine used in Thailand contained strains common to that part of the world. Participants in the North American study were men who have sex with men and uninfected partners of HIV-positive people. In Thailand, volunteers were uninfected intravenous drug users. Two-thirds of the North American volunteers were given the vaccine,

and the rest received a placebo. In Thailand, half the group received the vaccine and half were given a placebo. The four-year trial ended in 2002.

The trial results were reported on February 23, 2003. Unfortunately, AIDSvax was determined to be a failure, as the comparison of those who received the vaccine versus those receiving a placebo demonstrated a meager 3.8% reduction in new HIV infections in the vaccine population. This result is statistically insignificant. Surprisingly, Asians and blacks who received the vaccine displayed an astounding 67% lower rate of infection than their racial counterparts who received the placebo. Considerable debate has arisen concerning these latter observations. Was this a statistical fluke? Or did AIDSvax display demographically specific protection, and if so, why?

Although health officials and AIDS activists are hopeful, scientists are divided over when and which experimental vaccines should be approved for full-scale testing. Some favor trying any promising vaccine while others advise waiting until the vaccine is completely understood before testing it. The results of the AIDSvax trial could sway the argument toward the latter camp.

One potential problem with AIDSvax, and perhaps a partial explanation of the poor overall results, is that previous tests indicated that it boosted only one part of the immune system—the component of the immune system responsible for antibody production. It is generally believed that a truly effective anti-HIV vaccine must boost another part of the immune system—the killer T cells that destroy virus-infected cells. Some experts consider the vaccine a long shot, but others point out that a failed vaccine does not mean that the experiment failed. Negative results can teach researchers what not to do in the future.

Vaccine Research Center

In 2000 the Dale and Betty Bumpers Vaccine Research Center (VRC) opened on the NIH campus in Bethesda, Maryland. The $34 million facility is overseen by Anthony Fauci and brings together private companies and federal agencies to research, develop, and produce vaccines. Though VRC is not exclusively devoted to HIV research and will eventually begin efforts to develop vaccines for other diseases, VRC director Gary Nabel says HIV is a first target for the facility, which had $40 million in funding in 2002.

The first testing at VRC began in October 2001 and is a study of VRC-001-VP, a DNA vaccine that contains tiny amounts of reengineered HIV DNA. The clinical trial of VRC-001-VP involves volunteers who are not necessarily at risk for HIV infection and seeks to answer questions about how the immune system responds to the vaccine and the best timing for administering second and third doses of the vaccine.

The results were encouraging and demonstrated that the vaccine was safe, well-tolerated by the volunteers, and could induce immune responses. Beginning in December 2003, a larger clinical trial of the vaccine began. The encouraging results from the trial prompted a larger, ongoing clinical trial, which began in January 2005.

While most researchers are optimistic that an effective vaccine will be developed, many believe it may take as long as ten years to perfect a vaccine. As of 2005, researchers at the VRC believe that more than one vaccine formulation, or a vaccine that works two ways—to boost immunity provided by T cells and to produce antibodies to attach to HIV and mark it for destruction—may be necessary to provide complete protection.

A Dissenting View on Why There Is No Vaccine

A small group of researchers who call themselves the Group for the Scientific Reappraisal of the HIV/AIDS Hypothesis dispute the view widely held by the rest of the world's scientific community, namely that AIDS is caused by HIV. The two champions of this very controversial view are Peter Duesberg, who discovered the first cancer-related gene in 1970 and is a professor of molecular and cell biology at the University of California, Berkeley, and Kary Mullis, winner of the 1993 Nobel Prize in chemistry. Duesberg and Mullis disagree on exactly what causes AIDS, but they do agree that HIV is *not* the cause. In *Inventing the AIDS Virus* (Washington, DC: Regnery, 1996), Duesberg observed that despite huge efforts—more than one hundred thousand research papers published and $35 billion in taxpayer dollars spent—the HIV/AIDS hypothesis has failed to produce any public health benefits.

Duesberg bases his hotly disputed, highly controversial hypothesis, in part, on the fact that existing theories concerning the cause of AIDS rely on epidemiological, or circumstantial, evidence—that HIV is found in all people who have AIDS—and not on scientific proof that directly connects HIV with AIDS. If an infectious agent caused AIDS, Duesberg argues, it would exhibit five distinct qualities:

1. It would spread randomly between the sexes.

2. AIDS would appear quickly, in a matter of weeks or months instead of years.

3. Active and plentiful HIV microbes would be identifiable in all cases.

4. Cells would decrease or be impaired to the extent that the immune system could not replace them.

5. There would be a logical and consistent pattern of symptoms in AIDS patients.

Duesberg's reasoning is compelling to some: none of these qualities has been observed with HIV. Infection in men is far more common than in women, though this is changing; the onset of AIDS can take up to eleven years; the virus is difficult to isolate; cells in AIDS patients are replaced; and symptoms vary among patients.

Duesberg's detractors contend that the overwhelming body of research links HIV to AIDS. Even some of the critics, however, still agree with his basic observation: because more than twenty years have passed since AIDS was first described and research has failed to substantially change the fate of people with HIV/AIDS, new paths of investigation may be in order.

CHAPTER 7
PEOPLE WITH HIV/AIDS

Staggeringly large numbers of people are afflicted with HIV/AIDS in the United States. An increasing proportion of the population lives with HIV infection. By the early 2000s more Americans than ever before were likely to know someone affected by HIV or AIDS. Even people who live in remote geographic areas and do not believe they are personally at risk of acquiring HIV are aware of the epidemic from ongoing public health education campaigns, reports in the media, school health programs, and health and social service agencies dedicated to improving community awareness of HIV/AIDS.

PUBLIC FIGURES WITH HIV/AIDS

Perhaps one of the most famous HIV-infected people in the world is Earvin "Magic" Johnson, an internationally known former basketball player for the Los Angeles Lakers. When Johnson announced his HIV infection in September 1991, the world was shocked. He had no idea he was infected until he received the results of a routine physical examination for life insurance. Johnson freely admitted that prior to his marriage he had unprotected, and, in retrospect, unsafe, sexual contact with numerous women. He has no idea who transmitted the virus to him. The possibility exists that, however unknowingly, he passed the virus on to a subsequent sexual partner, who passed it on to someone else, and so on.

To many, Johnson became a hero for his courage and his immediate public acknowledgment of his HIV status. He became an HIV/AIDS spokesperson and began working in prevention programs. In 1991 Johnson started the Magic Johnson Foundation, which seeks to find funding and establish community-based education and social and health programs (including HIV/AIDS awareness) in inner-city communities and has given millions of dollars in grants to these causes. He was even named to the President's Commission on AIDS, from which he eventually resigned, frustrated with the lack of progress in

HIV/AIDS efforts by the administration of then-President George H. W. Bush.

Despite his active, well-publicized efforts to increase awareness and prevention of HIV/AIDS, some people considered him anything but a hero because his highly visible, promiscuous lifestyle sent the wrong message to the millions of young people who admired him.

In September 1992, one year after Johnson announced his retirement from professional basketball, he indicated that he was returning to basketball on a limited basis. He played on the U.S. "Dream Team" in the 1992 Olympics, assisting the team in its successful bid for the Gold Medal. Johnson benched himself at the start of the 1993–1994 season when he cut himself in a preseason game, terrifying some of his fellow players. While some players feared infection, others worried that they should not play against Johnson with full force; after all, he was a man with a fatal disease. Johnson came back again for the 1995–1996 season, helping his team reach the play-offs, and continues to play basketball with the Magic Johnson All-Stars Team. He shows others, as one observer notes, that HIV infection is not something you die of; it is something you live with.

In 1992 former tennis star Arthur Ashe announced that he had become infected with HIV from a blood transfusion in the mid-1980s during a heart bypass operation. His was not a voluntary announcement, but one made necessary when the news media discovered his HIV infection and threatened to announce it before he did. Ashe was reluctant to make his condition public, fearing the effect on his five-year-old daughter. He maintained that because he did not have a public responsibility, he should have been allowed to maintain his privacy. He died in 1994.

Greg Louganis, another athlete, was diagnosed with HIV infection in 1988. The Olympic gold medalist diver announced his HIV status after the 1992 Olympics, when he hit his head on the diving board during competition. Though his injury was not serious, it did result in an open wound. Today, Louganis is a television and movie actor, the published author of two books, and an advocate of safe sexual practices, since he attributes his HIV infection to unsafe sexual behavior.

Mary Fisher, a heterosexual and nondrug user who contracted HIV from her husband, stood before her peers at the 1992 Republican Convention and announced that she was infected with HIV. A former television producer and assistant to President Gerald R. Ford, she said she considered her announcement part of her contribution to the fight against HIV/AIDS. The wealthy, attractive, and well-educated Fisher was among the first women to publicly dispel the image that, unfortunately, still comes to mind when many people think of HIV/AIDS: homosexual, poor, drug-addicted, and lacking access to support systems or adequate medical care and housing.

Puerto Rican-born Esteban De Jesus became the world lightweight boxing champion in 1976 by beating Itshimatsu Suzuki of Japan. Five years prior to this fight, De Jesus had gained world attention by beating the legendary Roberto Duran, the then newly crowned lightweight champion, in a non-title bout. He retired from boxing with a stellar record of fifty-seven wins (thirty-two by knockout) and five losses. Following his retirement, De Jesus was convicted of murder in the death of a man allegedly in a drug-related dispute. While in prison, he was diagnosed with AIDS. In a humanitarian gesture, Puerto Rican governor Rafael Hernández Colón pardoned De Jesus in 1990. He died one month later.

Another sports celebrity who succumbed to AIDS was NASCAR race car driver Tim Richmond. Born on July 7, 1955, Richmond died of AIDS-related complications on August 13, 1989, at age thirty-four. During his heyday on the NASCAR race circuit in the 1980s, Richmond became one of the circuit's premier drivers. Richmond was well known for his expensive tastes in food and drink and for his "playboy" lifestyle. Whether his lifestyle contributed to his illness is conjecture. Nonetheless, by the end of the 1986 racing season, Richmond had become noticeably ill. He was diagnosed with AIDS that same year. He was able to race again in 1987, but soon thereafter his health deteriorated precipitously. During another attempted comeback in 1988, when his illness was still unpublicized, Richmond faced the hostility and innuendo of his fellow drivers, who, guessing the nature of the illness, speculated about his sexual orientation and the possibility of drug abuse. In response, Richmond filed a defamation of character lawsuit against NASCAR. He subsequently withdrew the lawsuit to avoid making his condition public. Richmond ultimately retired from competitive racing and lived in seclusion with his mother until his death. After his death,

as news of his affliction and the treatment he received from his fellow drivers and NASCAR became public, many people were outraged at the NASCAR organization, which has yet to apologize.

Actress Amanda Blake, best known for her nineteen-year role as Long Branch Saloon owner/operator Kitty Russell on the popular television series *Gunsmoke*, died in 1989 from throat cancer complicated by a type of AIDS-related viral hepatitis. Long a passionate supporter of animal rights, she was seminal in the founding of the Performing Animal Welfare Society (PAWS). Indeed, it is thought that she was infected with HIV during a PAWS-related trip to Africa.

Actor Brad Davis was another victim of AIDS. He was best known for his role in the 1978 movie *Midnight Express*, for which he received a Golden Globe award. He died of AIDS in 1991, after allegedly contracting the infection as a result of his cocaine abuse a decade earlier. His widow, Susan Bluestein, has continued to campaign for AIDS causes.

Actor Anthony Perkins, who is best known for his role as Norman Bates in the classic Alfred Hitchcock film *Psycho*, also died of AIDS. Forever typecast by that performance, Perkins was in fact an accomplished film and stage actor. He was bisexual and had relationships with a number of men including dancer Rudolf Nureyev (who also died of AIDS). Shortly before his death in 1992, Perkins commented in a press release about a *National Enquirer* article that revealed his AIDS-positive status by saying, "I have learned more about love, selflessness and human understanding from the people I have met in this great adventure in the world of AIDS than I ever did in the cutthroat, competitive world in which I spent my life." Perkin's widow, Berry Berenson, was one of the passengers on American Airlines Flight 11, which was hijacked and crashed into the World Trade Center North Tower on September 11, 2001.

Another movie star who succumbed to AIDS was Rock Hudson. Indeed, Hudson was the first major U.S. celebrity known to have died from AIDS. His death was especially noteworthy, given his status in the 1950s as the quintessential rugged, all-American male. Despite his many movie roles as a straight man, Hudson was homosexual, a fact that was covered up by movie studios. His 1955 marriage to studio employee Phyllis Gates (which ended in divorce in 1958) is thought to have been a studio-orchestrated attempt to cover up his sexual orientation. Hudson died in 1985 at the age of fifty-nine.

African-American rap star Eric Wright, whose moniker was Eazy-E, rose to fame as one of the members of the Compton, California-based group N.W.A. (Niggaz with Attitude). Using the money from illegal drug sales, Eazy-E had founded Ruthless Records. Soon after, he recruited

Ice Cube, Dr. Dre, MC Ren, DJ Yella, and Arabian Prince to form N.W.A. The group's second album, *Straight Outta Compton*, which was released in 1988, became hugely popular. Following the dissolution of N.W.A., Eazy-E went on to have a successful solo career. In 1995 he entered the hospital for treatment of what he thought was asthma. But he was diagnosed with AIDS, which he did not hesitate in confirming. He died soon after. Eazy-E is now regarded as being one of the influential founders of the style of music known as gangsta rap. Every year, the city of Compton celebrates his life by observing Eazy-E Day.

Another music icon who died of AIDS was Freddie Mercury, the lead vocalist of the British rock band Queen. His more than three-octave vocal range and operatic compositional approach to rock resulted in classic hits such as "Bohemian Rhapsody," "Somebody to Love," and "We Are the Champions." The video that was made for the 1975 release of "Bohemian Rhapsody" is considered by some music insiders to be one of the seminal influences that spurred the popularity of music videos. Mercury was well known for his bisexuality, which for some years was promiscuous, and the extravagance and hedonism of his lifestyle. His diagnosis and deteriorating physical condition were kept private. Indeed, his eventual announcement that he had AIDS was made only one day before his death in 1991.

Elizabeth Glaser, wife of Paul Michael Glaser (one of the stars of the 1970s television series *Starsky and Hutch*), was galvanized to cofound the Pediatric AIDS Foundation in 1988 (now called the Elizabeth Glaser Pediatric AIDS Foundation) following the discovery that she and her and Paul Michael's children, Ariel and Jake, were all infected with HIV. She originally contracted the virus from contaminated blood administered during pregnancy, but she was unaware of her illness until much later, already having unwittingly passed it to her children. In the ensuing years she became a vocal AIDS activist. The foundation that is her legacy contributes more than one million dollars annually to pediatric AIDS research. Elizabeth Glaser died in 1994. Her daughter Ariel died before Elizabeth, at age seven; her son Jake still lives with the disease; and her husband continues to raise money and AIDS awareness through her foundation.

Finally, in a list of examples that is by no means complete, prolific and influential science fiction author Isaac Asimov contracted HIV from infected blood given to him in a transfusion during heart bypass surgery in 1983. He died on April 6, 1992, of heart and renal failure that were complications of AIDS.

OLDER PEOPLE WITH HIV/AIDS

In "AIDS among Persons Aged 50 Years and Over—United States, 1991–1996" (*Morbidity and Mortality Weekly Report*, vol. 47, no. 2, 1998), the Centers for Disease Control and Prevention (CDC) reports that most older people infected with HIV early in the epidemic were typically infected through contaminated blood or blood products. Through 1989 only 1% of HIV/AIDS cases of people ages thirteen to forty-nine was due to contaminated blood. But in that same period 6% of cases of people fifty to fifty-nine, 28% of cases of people sixty to sixty-nine, and 64% of cases of those seventy and older resulted from contaminated blood or blood products.

In 1985 changes introduced to improve the safety of the nation's blood supply, including routine screening of blood donations for HIV, sharply reduced the risk of contracting the virus from contaminated blood or blood products. Subsequently, the proportion of people age fifty and over who acquired HIV from other types of exposure increased. Although male to male sexual contact and intravenous drug use remain the primary means by which HIV is transmitted among all age groups in the United States, heterosexual transmission of HIV is steadily increasing in people more than fifty years old.

HIV/AIDS Cases among People Age Forty-Five and Over

Approximately 11 to 15% of AIDS cases reported in the United States occur in people over age fifty, according to the CDC. This proportion did not vary much between 1991 and 1999. But it is expected to increase as HIV-infected people of all ages live longer as a result of effective drug therapy and other advances in medical treatment.

To December 2003, 150,063 cases of AIDS in people over age forty-five have been reported to the CDC. Among these reported cases, more than 80% were men, approximately 16% were women, almost 40% were African-American men and women, and approximately 17% were Hispanic men and women. More than three-quarters of AIDS cases reported in people over age sixty-five were from large metropolitan areas.

HIV Testing for Those over Age Fifty

Many older adults do not seek routine screening for HIV infection because they do not believe they are at risk of acquiring HIV. Among women older than fifty, the absence of the risk of pregnancy may lead to a false sense of security and the mistaken belief that they are at less risk for sexually transmitted diseases, including HIV. HIV-infected people age fifty and over may not be tested promptly for HIV infection. As a result, opportunities to start these patients on therapies quickly in order to slow the progression of the disease are often lost. The failure to test or the late testing of older patients may be because:

- Physicians are less apt to look for HIV in people of this age group.

- Some opportunistic AIDS illnesses that occur in older people, such as encephalopathy and wasting disease, have similar symptoms to other diseases associated with aging, such as Alzheimer's disease, depression, and malignancies.

It is vitally important to overcome older adults' reluctance to seek testing and other delays to diagnosis because recent research shows that age speeds the progression of HIV to AIDS and blunts CD4 response to highly active antiretroviral therapy. Equally important is continuing research to improve treatment of HIV-infected older adults and development of effective education programs to prevent infection in this population.

LIVING WITH HIV/AIDS

In order to gain a more complete view of the impact of HIV/AIDS, it is important to understand the psychosocial and emotional consequences of diagnosis with a potentially fatal disease.

A Frightening Diagnosis

In his introduction to *When Someone Close Has AIDS* (Washington, DC: National Institute of Mental Health, 1989), National Institute of Mental Health director Lewis L. Judd writes about the meaning of the diagnosis of AIDS. It means not only a shortened life, but also one that is "marred by chronic fatigue, loss of appetite and weight, frequent hospitalizations, AIDS dementia, and debilitating bouts of illness from unusual infections." The person diagnosed with HIV/AIDS also feels anger, confusion, depression, isolation, and hopelessness, which can also affect those around him or her who are often unprepared for the suffering they witness.

Judd advises that people diagnosed with HIV/AIDS need reassurance from friends and relatives that they will not be abandoned or isolated. He also recommends that those around HIV/AIDS patients encourage them to pursue hobbies, work as long as they can, and engage in social activities. He warns that caring for someone with AIDS is physically and emotionally exhausting and calls for inner strength, as well as the caregivers' coming to terms with their own feelings about the illness.

Coping with Discrimination

Unlike people diagnosed with other terminal or catastrophic illnesses such as cancer or multiple sclerosis, people with HIV/AIDS often confront the social isolation and discrimination that accompany a stigmatized status. Many people think of HIV/AIDS as a disease of homosexual men and drug users and believe that these people

brought HIV/AIDS on themselves. Some still believe that AIDS is divine retribution for an "immoral lifestyle." Fear of unfavorable judgment keeps many infected individuals from disclosing their HIV infection to others, even friends and loved ones. Others simply do not want the pity that is often extended to people with fatal conditions. Still others worry that friends and family, fearing infection, will abandon them.

Under the Americans with Disabilities Act (ADA) of 1990, people infected with HIV and those diagnosed with AIDS are considered disabled and as such are subject to the antidiscrimination provisions of this landmark legislation. As a result, employers generally may not ask job applicants if they are HIV infected or have AIDS, nor can they require an HIV test of prospective employees. The only exceptions to this provision are those employers who can demonstrate that such questions or testing are job related and absolutely necessary for the employer to conduct business.

More importantly, the ADA requires employers to make "reasonable accommodations" for disabled employees. Reasonable accommodation is an adjustment to a job or modification of the responsibilities or work environment that will enable the worker with a disability to gain equal employment opportunity. Examples include flexible work schedules to allow for medical appointments, treatments, and counseling and the provision of additional unpaid leave.

THE STIGMA OF AIDS. In 1995 the Department of Sociology and Social Work at Fort Hays State University, Kansas, conducted a survey to find how knowledge and mode of transmission affected opinions of people with AIDS. In "The Stigma of AIDS: Persons with AIDS and Social Distance" (*Deviant Behavior*, October–December 1995), J. J. Leiker, D. E. Taub, and J. Gast write that as HIV/AIDS knowledge increases, people tend to attach less stigma to the disease.

According to the survey, respondents attached the least stigma to those infected by blood transfusions. The greatest stigma was attached to exposures from male to male sexual behavior and intravenous drug use. Survey participants who considered themselves homophobic (having a fear of or aversion to homosexuality) attached more of a stigma to people with AIDS than those who did not feel they were homophobic. People who labeled themselves "religious" attached less stigma to those infected through blood transfusions.

More than two decades after the first diagnoses of AIDS and widespread public health and community education efforts to inform people about HIV infection and prevent the spread of HIV, ignorance and misunderstanding of HIV/AIDS persist. Health educators and HIV/AIDS activists stress the importance of intensified, ongoing education to destigmatize people affected by HIV/AIDS and prevent discrimination. Reducing the stigma associated with HIV/AIDS may also encourage individuals to get tested and, for those who are infected, begin treatment as soon as possible.

In "Will Focus on Terrorism Overshadow the Fight against AIDS?" (*Journal of the American Medical Association*, November 7, 2001), Rebecca Voelker observes that after more than two decades the stigma associated with AIDS should have dropped to very low, barely detectable levels. Unfortunately, it has not diminished as expected. Researcher Lisanne Francis Brown of the Tulane University School of Public Health feels it is important to identify strategies to reduce stigma since it "undermines efforts to combat the epidemic at every level."

Dealing with Emotions

Not unexpectedly, anger and depression are natural and common reactions to discovering that one has an HIV infection. While experts stress the importance of recognizing and expressing anger and depression, if these feelings become all-consuming, they can prevent health- and life-improving actions. Many people with HIV/AIDS admit that sharing feelings with friends and family members and participating in support groups ease anguish and help generate more positive attitudes and actions.

Many HIV/AIDS sufferers report that the most difficult thing they had to do after being diagnosed with HIV was to inform people in their present or recent past whom they might have exposed to the virus. If the patient is unable to do this, a physician or public health official can notify present or former sexual partners without revealing the infected person's name.

Early Medication Improves Outlook

The earlier a person learns of his or her infection, the earlier he or she can begin medical treatment to suppress the virus's destructive growth, delay the onset of AIDS symptoms, and extend life. Along with antiretroviral drugs there are medications that fight the life-threatening opportunistic infections that eventually afflict most people who are HIV infected. Although these drugs cannot cure HIV infection, they have been shown to keep HIV/AIDS patients healthy and symptom-free for increasingly longer periods.

Practicing Good Health Habits

Experts advise HIV-infected people to exercise and maintain a balanced diet with sufficient lean protein. Not only does exercise improve overall fitness and generate a sense of well-being, it also releases endorphins, which are natural substances produced by the brain that boost immunity, reduce stress, and elevate mood. People with HIV/AIDS are advised to avoid smoking, excessive alcohol consumption, and using illegal drugs, all of which can act to depress the immune system.

Stress Not a Factor?

In addition to new health concerns, people with HIV/AIDS must confront an altered identity. Those diagnosed with HIV infection must immediately reevaluate their life goals. For example, saving money for retirement or a new car may no longer seem important. HIV-infected individuals often lose their health insurance coverage and must consider saving money for future health care needs and/or meeting eligibility requirements for health care coverage from Medicaid, the government entitlement program. They also must confront fears and uncertainty about the future such as how to care and provide for children or other loved ones.

Interestingly, a study conducted by Ronald C. Kessler, a research scientist at the University of Michigan's Institute for Social Research, indicates that stressful life events do not appear to trigger the development of AIDS symptoms in HIV-positive men who are feeling healthy. The findings, released in 1992, still warrant discussion in 2005. The findings are based on a correlation between the health and psychological status of 980 gay men in Chicago who participated in two studies from 1984 to 1987 ("The National Multicenter AIDS Cohort Study" and "The Coping and Change Study," both funded by the National Institute of Mental Health). The results of these landmark studies are considered to refute conclusively the hypothesis that stress plays a pivotal role in triggering the development of AIDS among people with HIV infection.

The data, collected twice each year, included the incidence and nature of stressful life events and the development of three HIV symptoms: fevers lasting longer than two weeks, bacterial infections of the throat and mouth (oral thrush), and declines of 25% or more in the number of T cells. One aim of the study was to investigate the findings of an earlier unpublished study that had found that HIV-positive men who were close to others with AIDS or people dying from AIDS often experienced a sudden onset of symptoms themselves.

The University of Michigan study measured the impact of twenty-four other serious stresses on health, such as job loss, death of a parent, and mortgage foreclosure, and found no consistent relationship between stressful events and the onset of HIV symptoms. Kessler does find that men who were grieving for deceased loved ones were more likely to suffer a decline in T cells and develop other symptoms, but he does not believe that this was an effect of a stressful event. Instead, it is more likely that those who had an onset of symptoms after friends died from AIDS were probably in the same group who were infected early in the epidemic.

HOUSING PROBLEMS

The difficulty in finding affordable and appropriate housing can be an acute crisis for people living with HIV/AIDS. HIV-infected people need more than just a safe shelter that provides protection and comfort; they may also require a base from which to receive services, care, and support. While adherence to complicated medical regimens is challenging for many HIV-infected people, for some homeless people it is nearly impossible.

While some individuals are homeless when they acquire HIV infection, others lose their homes when they are no longer able to hold jobs or cannot afford to pay for health care and housing costs. The National AIDS Housing Coalition reports that, by 2006, 50% of the estimated 886,575 people who will be living with HIV/AIDS will require some form of housing assistance.

The Department of Veterans Affairs reports that as many as one-third to one-half of all people with HIV/AIDS are either homeless or at great risk of becoming homeless due to their illness, a lack of income or other resources, and a weak support network. Several studies indicate that approximately 30% of all people with HIV in acute care hospitals (at a cost of more than $1,000 per day) are hospitalized not because they require the medical services available in the hospital, but simply because no community-based residential program will take them. According to the National Coalition for the Homeless, 1999 data show that more than 30% of HIV-infected people had become homeless since learning they were infected.

In 1990 the Department of Housing and Urban Development established a federal program specifically intended to meet the housing needs of people with HIV/AIDS. Congress established the program because the housing resources available at that time were not meeting the needs of people with AIDS, who, due to discrimination, had difficulties obtaining suitable housing and the supportive services that they required. The program Housing Opportunities for Persons with AIDS (HOPWA) was established under the National Affordable Housing Act of 1990 (PL 101–625). HOPWA began in 1992, and between that fiscal year (FY) and FY 2001, Congress allotted more than $1.5 billion for the program. In FY 2002 an additional $277 million was allocated, an increase of $19 million over the preceding year. FY 2003 funding was $290.1 million, about $13 million more than in 2002.

SUICIDE

Depression is a common psychiatric problem among patients who are seriously ill with HIV/AIDS. While this is a normal grief response, the combination of alienation, hopelessness, guilt, and lack of self-esteem can lead some to contemplate and plan for suicide in search of lost dignity and control. Others counter that the real dignity is in seeing the disease to the end. Those who encourage people with HIV/AIDS to "stick it out" often see the disease as becoming increasingly manageable with drugs and improved treatment techniques.

Several factors make HIV/AIDS patients more likely to commit suicide: they know they are certain to die sooner than they expected and chances are it will be emotionally and physically painful; they may lose their jobs, their insurance, or their homes; and they may be ostracized from society. Researchers find that factors that have a considerable impact on the quality of life include security, family, love, pleasurable activity, and freedom from pain and suffering and from debilitating disease. AIDS patients may lose all of these. For some, suicide seems like a reasonable alternative; it offers an end to pain and suffering, insecurity, self-pity, dependency, and hopelessness.

Euthanasia in the Netherlands

Euthanasia (ending the lives—for reasons of mercy—of those who are hopelessly ill or injured) and physician-assisted suicide are other unnatural deaths that are often requested by patients themselves. Euthanasia is illegal in the United States (although Oregon's controversial "Death with Dignity Act" allows physicians to help severely ill patients commit suicide if they meet certain criteria). In the Netherlands, however, euthanasia was officially legalized in 2001. While technically illegal prior to this, euthanasia had in fact been tolerated and studied in that country for many years. A 1995 study sponsored by Amsterdam's Municipal Health Service found that 22% of the 131 men with AIDS studied died from requested euthanasia or physician-assisted suicide. Among the 22%, physicians reported that 72% would have died within one month. The survey also found that the likelihood of euthanasia/physician-assisted suicide increased with the duration of survival after AIDS diagnosis and among those over the age of forty.

The authors of the Amsterdam study note that because AIDS patients usually know for many years that they are infected with HIV, they have time to discuss their condition and the possibility of euthanasia. Many of these people, explains a counselor of AIDS patients, choose euthanasia because it gives them the opportunity to die on their own terms.

The Physician's Role

In 1994–95 Lee R. Slome et al. ("Physician-Assisted Suicide and Patients with Human Immunodeficiency Virus Disease," *New England Journal of Medicine*, vol. 336, no. 6, 1997) surveyed all 228 physicians in the Community Consortium in the San Francisco Bay area of California. The researchers wanted to find out whether physicians were participating—or would be willing to participate to

TABLE 7.1

TABLE 7.2

Characteristics of physicians responding to 1990 and 1995 surveys on physician-assisted suicide and HIV

Characteristic	1990 (N=69)	1995 (N=118)
	Percent	
Sex		
Male	81	73
Female	19	27
Race or ethnic group		
White	97	89
Black	0	4
Hispanic	1	3
Asian or Pacific Islander	2	4
Sexual orientation		
Homosexual or bisexual	55	36
Heterosexual	45	64
Martial status		
Married	33	47
Unmarried but in a relationship	36	32
Unmarried and not in a relationship	30	21
Religion		
Protestant	26	17
Catholic	13	12
Jewish	36	30
Other	25	41
Total no. of patients with AIDS		
0	9	0
1–20	4	3
21–40	7	8
41–60	7	4
61–80	9	5
>80	63	78

Note: Because of rounding, percentages do not sum to 100.

SOURCE: Lee R. Slome, Thomas F. Mitchell, Edwin Charlesbois, et al., "Characteristics of Respondents to the 1990 and 1995 Surveys," in "Physician-Assisted Suicide and Patients with Human Immunodeficiency Virus Disease," in the *New England Journal of Medicine*, vol. 336, no. 6, February 6, 1997

Physician responses to case vignette in 1990 and 1995

Question and response	1990 no. (%)	1995 no. (%)
How likely would you be to prescribe a lethal dose of medication for Tom?[a]		
Very unlikely	20 (29)	18 (16)
Unlikely	20 (29)	19 (17)
Neither likely nor unlikely	9 (13)	22 (19)
Likely	13 (19)	47 (41)
Very likely	6 (9)	8 (7)
If Tom was adamant about getting assistance in committing suicide, what course of action would you take?[b]		
Refuse his request	10 (14)	18 (16)
Talk him out of it	16 (23)	12 (11)
Hospitalize him as a danger to himself	2 (3)	1 (1)
Refer him to a mental health professional	41 (59)	50 (45)
Refer him to a suicide-prevention program	4 (6)	5 (5)
Refer him to clergy	11 (16)	17 (15)
Refer him to another physician	1 (1)	8 (7)
Refer him to the Hemlock Society	32 (46)	42 (38)
Grant his request	24 (35)	56 (51)

Note: Only the physicians who responded to question about the case vignette are included.
[a] There were 68 respondents in 1990 and 114 in 1995.
[b] There were 69 respondents in 1990 and 110 in 1995. More than one response per physician was possible.

SOURCE: Lee R. Slome, Thomas F. Mitchell, Edwin Charlesbois, et al., "Physician Responses to Case Vignette in 1990 and 1995," in "Physician-Assisted Suicide and Patients with Human Immunodeficiency Virus Disease," in the *New England Journal of Medicine*, vol. 336, no. 6, February 6, 1997

any extent—in physician-assisted suicide, which was defined as providing a patient with a sufficient dose of narcotics to kill him- or herself.

The physicians who treated HIV patients were told in the anonymous, self-administered survey that the fictitious patient, Tom, was a severely ill, mentally incompetent thirty-year-old man facing imminent death. A similar survey had been conducted in 1990. Compared to the 1990 respondents, the 118 physicians who responded to the 1995 survey were more racially diverse, more likely to be heterosexual, and more apt to have a large number of AIDS patients. (See Table 7.1.)

Of the 1995 respondents, 48% said they would be likely or very likely to grant Tom's initial request for physician-assisted suicide, compared with 28% of the 1990 respondents. When asked what they would do if Tom was insistent about his request, 51% of the 1995 respondents said they would grant it, compared with 35%

of the 1990 respondents. The 1995 physicians (11%) were also less likely than the 1990 physicians (23%) to try to talk the patient out of his request. (See Table 7.2.)

Slome et al. also asked the physician respondents to estimate the number of times they had helped an AIDS patient commit suicide. Of the 117 who responded, about half (53%) indicated that they had prescribed a fatal dose of medication at least once to an AIDS patient. (Figure 7.1 shows the distribution of the number of patients assisted in suicide.) The researchers note that this number was surprisingly high, given the possible legal and ethical consequences of such an action.

The researchers concluded that:

- The survey suggests an increasing acceptance among physicians of assisted suicide.

- A physician's sexual orientation (homosexual or bisexual) is positively related to his or her willingness to assist in suicide, although sexual orientation is only one of four factors affecting the doctors' decision. (See Table 7.1 for other factors or characteristics of respondents.)

- Some doctors consider their assistance to be psychological intervention rather than a means of facilitating death; that is, the medication allows patients to regain some of the control AIDS has taken away.

FIGURE 7.1

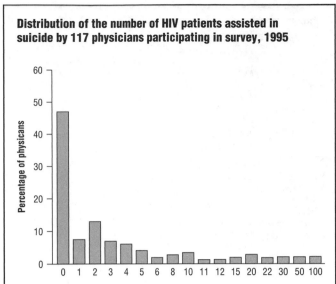

Distribution of the number of HIV patients assisted in suicide by 117 physicians participating in survey, 1995

SOURCE: Lee R. Slome, Thomas F. Mitchell, Edwin Charlesbois, et al., "Distribution of the Number of Patients with HIV Assisted in Suicide by 117 Physicians Participating in Survey, 1995," in "Physician-Assisted Suicide and Patients with Human Immunodeficiency Virus Disease," in the *New England Journal of Medicine*, vol. 336, no. 6, February 6, 1997

During the 1990s there were heated debates, voter initiatives, and court decisions about the legalization of physician-assisted suicide. Only one U.S. state—Oregon—has legalized physician-assisted suicide; Oregon voters determined that the right to end one's own life is intensely personal and should not be forbidden by law. (Though attempts and acts of suicide are no longer subject to criminal prosecution in the United States, aiding a suicide is considered a criminal offense.)

Both the public and physicians themselves are divided about the issue of physician-assisted suicide. People who support the practice believe that doctors should make their skills available to patients to end anguish and suffering. Those who oppose physician-assisted suicide argue that better end-of-life care—effective pain management, emotional and spiritual support, and widespread education to reduce anxiety about dying—may reduce the frequency of requests for physician-assisted suicide. Opponents also fear that the legal right to assist suicide has the potential to be misused or abused and that such abuses might victimize already vulnerable populations.

CHAPTER 8
TESTING, PREVENTION, AND EDUCATION

HIV TESTING
Voluntary, Not Mandatory

Few issues about the HIV/AIDS epidemic have prompted more controversy than the use of antibody tests to identify people who are infected with HIV. Soon after the enzyme-linked immunosorbent assay test was developed and licensed in 1985, many public health officials supported testing in an attempt to change "undesirable" behaviors that were determining the course of the epidemic (such as male to male sexual contact [MTM] and intravenous drug use [IDU]). Those who favored testing claimed that if a person knew he or she was HIV-positive, the infected person would change his or her behavior. Others argued that aggressive public health education and carefully planned and implemented counseling would be more productive strategies to achieve the desired results, even if people did not know their HIV status.

In the early years of the epidemic, health care officials in the public and private sectors refrained from advocating mandatory testing; instead, they focused on HIV testing that would be performed by physicians for patients they believed to be at risk for infection. In 1990 the House of Delegates of the American Medical Association (AMA) voted to declare HIV/AIDS a sexually transmitted disease (STD). This designation allowed physicians more freedom to decide the conditions under which HIV testing should take place.

In the late 1980s, when the research community announced that HIV-infected, symptom-free people could receive early intervention with azidothymidine (also known as zidovudine) to slow the effects of the illness and delay the onset of *Pneumocystis carinii* pneumonia, the debate took another turn. Gay rights advocates, such as the Gay Men's Health Crisis Center in New York, began to encourage those at risk for HIV infection to get tested rather than discouraging testing, as the group

had previously done. In June 1997 the Center opened its own testing facility. This service continues in 2005 as part of the range of care and support services offered by the Michael Palm Center. The center also offers a twelve-week "harm reduction program" designed to curb risky behaviors such as substance abuse and unprotected sex. The intent of the program is to encourage people to change their risky behavior in a supportive atmosphere of care.

Another controversy surrounding testing concerns reporting HIV-positive patients by name. Every state is required to report AIDS cases. As of December 2003 forty-one states, American Samoa, Guam, the U.S. Mariana Islands, and the U.S. Virgin Islands had implemented HIV case surveillance using the same confidential system for name-based case reporting for both HIV infection and AIDS. (See Table 8.1.)

Only Connecticut and Oregon conduct pediatric surveillance. Washington State implements HIV reporting by patient name to enable public health follow-up; after services and referrals are offered, names are converted into codes. At least six states (California, Illinois, Maine, Maryland, Massachusetts, and Pennsylvania) and Puerto Rico are reporting cases of HIV infection using a coded identifier rather than patient name. In most other states HIV case reporting was under consideration, or regulations enabling HIV surveillance were expected to be implemented. As of 2003 thirty-six states reported pediatric AIDS statistics as part of their confidential surveillance programs.

Critics, including the American Civil Liberties Union, assail name reporting as an invasion of privacy that carries social and economic risks. They claim that any benefit that would result from reporting names could not override the negative consequences (such as ostracism and loss of jobs and health insurance) of being classified as infected. They

TABLE 8.1

Reported cases of HIV infection, by area of residence and age category, cumulative through 2003

Area of residence (date HIV reporting initiated)	2003 No.	Cumulative through 2003[a]		
		Adults or adolescents	Children (<13 years)	Total
Alabama (Jan. 1988)	501	6,065	45	6,110
Alaska (Feb. 1999)	39	277	2	279
Arizona (Jan. 1987)	510	5,343	56	5,399
Arkansas (July 1989)	183	2,290	21	2,311
Colorado (Nov. 1985)	365	6,295	28	6,323
Connecticut (July 1992)[b]	1	—	106	106
Florida (July 1997)[c]	5,467	31,191	306	31,497
Georgia (Dec. 2003)	52	502	13	515
Idaho (June 1986)	28	429	4	433
Indiana (July 1988)	336	3,985	46	4,031
Iowa (July 1998)	43	465	6	471
Kansas (July 1999)	93	1,120	14	1,134
Louisiana (Feb. 1993)	787	8,030	134	8,164
Michigan (April 1992)	548	6,196	129	6,325
Minnesota (Oct. 1985)	225	3,256	35	3,291
Mississippi (Aug. 1988)	354	4,548	54	4,602
Missouri (Oct. 1987)	467	4,968	51	5,019
Nebraska (Sept. 1995)	48	604	8	612
Nevada (Feb. 1992)	221	3,488	22	3,510
New Jersey (Jan. 1992)	1,361	16,382	423	16,805
New Mexico (Jan. 1998)	71	775	3	778
New York (June 2000)	8,403	34,194	1,868	36,062
North Carolina (Feb. 1990)	1,315	12,453	133	12,586
North Dakota (Jan. 1988)	2	84	1	85
Ohio (June 1990)	786	7,438	89	7,527
Oklahoma (June 1988)	206	2,674	30	2,704
Pennsylvania (Oct. 2002)[d]	2,665	3,258	45	3,303
South Carolina (Feb. 1986)	539	7,527	108	7,635
South Dakota (Jan. 1988)	18	224	4	228
Tennessee (Jan. 1992)	696	6,812	85	6,897
Texas (Jan. 1999)[e]	4,292	18,023	375	18,398
Utah (April 1989)	96	687	11	698
Virginia (July 1989)	723	9,555	81	9,636
West Virginia (Jan. 1989)	92	707	6	713
Wisconsin (Nov. 1985)	172	2,508	32	2,540
Wyoming (June 1989)	10	95	1	96
Subtotal	31,715	212,448	4,375	216,823
U.S. dependencies, possessions, and associated nations				
American Samoa (Aug. 2001)	0	1	0	1
Guam (March 2000)	0	60	0	60
Northern Mariana Islands (Oct. 2001)	0	5	0	5
Puerto Rico (Jan. 2003)	951	965	10	975
Virgin Islands, U.S. (Dec. 1988)	25	243	6	249
Persons reported from states with confidential name-based HIV infection reporting, who were residents of other states	421	1,981	151	2,132
Total[f]	33,301	216,486	4,579	221,065

Note: Includes only persons with HIV infection that has not progressed to AIDS. Includes data from 37 states and from U.S. dependencies, possessions, and independent nations in free association with the United States.

[a]Includes persons with a diagnosis of HIV infection, reported from the beginning of the epidemic through 2003.

[b]Connecticut has confidential name-based HIV infection reporting only for pediatric cases.

[c]Florida (since July 1997) has had confidential name-based HIV infection reporting only for new diagnoses.

[d]Pennsylvania (October 2002) implemented confidential name-based HIV infection reporting only in areas outside the city of Philadelphia.

[e]Texas (February 1994 through December 1998) reported only pediatric HIV infection cases.

[f]Includes 812 persons reported from areas with confidential name-based HIV infection reporting, but whose area of residence is unknown. Includes 7 children reported from Oregon prior to the change in 2001 from name-based HIV infection reporting for pediatric cases to code-based reporting for all persons with HIV infection.

SOURCE: "Table 16. Reported Cases of HIV Infection (Not AIDS), by Area of Residence and Age Category, Cumulative through 2003—41 Areas with Confidential Name-Based HIV Infection Reporting," in *HIV/AIDS Surveillance Report: Cases of HIV infection and AIDS in the United States, 2003*, vol. 15, Centers for Disease Control and Prevention, 2004, http://www.cdc.gov/hiv/stats/2003surveillanceReport.pdf (accessed July 18, 2005)

add that name reporting discourages those at risk for HIV from coming forward to seek testing and timely treatment.

The American Medical Association and other advocates for reporting patients by name claim that it is essential for contact tracing, or partner notification, so that others who may have been infected will obtain treatment and other services. In Iowa, before name-reporting legislation had been adopted, John Katz, the STD/HIV program manager for the state's Department of Public Health, claimed that it was virtually impossible to determine trends without name reporting. Patients have repeat tests, and tests are performed to verify the analytical accuracy of testing labs. An anonymous system can confuse test results when testing is repeated in this way. Katz stated that not using name reporting "essentially leaves us with . . . a big batch of nothing. We can tell how many positive tests have been reported, but I can't tell you how many human beings that represents."

Demographic data are used in states that do not require name reporting. During 1998 the Centers for Disease Control and Prevention (CDC) funded projects in Texas and Maryland that incorporated unique identifiers (the last four digits of the Social Security number, birth date, sex, and race), instead of names, for those tested. While the name-reporting debate continues, there is widespread agreement that testing is most effective if followed by counseling that completely explains the results and their consequences.

Counseling and Testing

Counseling and testing are important components of state and local HIV-prevention programs. Testing at publicly funded centers is free or available at nominal cost. In contrast, testing through a private physician can cost more than $200.

Each year the CDC conducts the world's largest telephone survey to track health risks in the United States. People between the ages of eighteen and sixty-five in forty-nine states and the District of Columbia respond to the telephone survey. Examination of the data from the 2000 Behavioral Risk Factor Surveillance System survey is typical of data obtained and, as of June 2005, represents the most current year for which HIV/AIDS data was obtained.

A median (half the states had more; half had less) of 45.7% of respondents reported having at least one HIV-antibody test; in 1998 a median of 40% of respondents had been tested for HIV. The 2000 survey found the proportions of those who had been tested for reasons other than donating blood ranged from a low of 35% in Minnesota to a high of 65.3% in the District of Columbia. Of those who had been tested for HIV, a median of 86.4% reported receiving the results of their last HIV test; less than one-third of those tested (the median was 32.3%) received post-HIV test counseling.

Contact Tracing/Partner Notification

A by-product of testing is contact tracing, or partner notification. When individuals test positive for HIV, health officials ask them to provide, with the promise of anonymity, the names of those with whom they have had sexual contact or shared needles. The CDC asks counselors to inform contacts if the patient is reluctant to do so and strongly endorses contact-tracing programs, but results vary. States struggling under the strain of numerous HIV/AIDS cases continue to support programs that encourage the infected people to notify partners on their own. Contact-tracing programs in states with fewer HIV/AIDS cases are more likely to contact partners. Many patients who have HIV or AIDS fear that the promises of confidentiality will be broken; others fear retribution from those they may have infected.

Increasingly, states are trying to expand contact-tracing programs of health departments that notify sexual partners exposed to the virus. As an example, since 1995 health department counselors in Missouri's partner notification system have received additional training in teaching skills to reduce risky behavior. CDC-funded demonstration projects such as the San Francisco Bay Area Partner Assistance, Information, and Referral Services, which began in 1998, are trying to determine whether aggressive, confidential partner notification will prove to be an effective HIV prevention measure.

Home Testing

Home HIV tests were developed in the mid-1980s but were opposed by the Food and Drug Administration (FDA) and some HIV/AIDS organizations and health care agencies. The FDA was concerned about telephone counseling for those who tested positive, the accuracy of the tests, and confidentiality. In 1996 the FDA reversed its position, deciding that despite its limitations, the benefits of home testing outweighed the risks.

The CDC claims that significant numbers of people have acquired HIV but do not know it. Many, say public health officials, are afraid of getting tested at a physician's office or public clinic because of the associated stigma. Some drug companies suggest that an HIV-antibody test that can be performed at home may be the only way some of these people will learn their HIV status and argue that more people will then take steps to get treatment and prevent spreading the infection.

Some home tests use saliva, which does not require a needle stick, and others use blood samples. When blood is tested, the patient draws a few drops of blood from a fingertip, places it on filter paper, and mails the paper to a company laboratory, which performs the standard HIV assay. If the results are positive, a confirmation test is performed. An HIV test kit called the Home Access Express HIV-1 Test System, manufactured by Home Access Health, which was approved by the FDA in 1996, remains the only HIV home test kit approved by the agency as of June 2005. Three days after the Home Access Express test kit is received by Home Access Health, results and counseling are available by calling a twenty-four-hour toll-free number and giving an identification code. Home Access claims a greater than 99.9% accuracy rate.

Critics of home testing say that news of HIV infection is not as easy to accept as the results of other in-home tests, such as those for pregnancy and cholesterol. They claim that most people cannot properly prepare themselves for the news that they have a life-threatening disease. They advocate expansion of current testing sites to include mobile vans, sports clubs, and other places that are not exclusively associated with HIV testing, but where in-person counseling could be provided.

Military Practices

The Department of Defense (DOD) regularly screens all members of the armed services and those seeking to join for HIV. Annual HIV testing is required of all personnel on active duty, as well as all members of the reserves and National Guard. In 1995, after two months of debate on Capitol Hill, federal legislators scrapped a discharge provision that would have forced the DOD to dismiss members of the military within six months of testing positive for HIV. Along with HIV infection, a number of chronic conditions, including cancer, asthma, diabetes, heart disease, or complications of pregnancy place troops on limited assignment, precluding them from overseas service or combat.

Debating the merits of permitting HIV-infected personnel to remain in the military, representative Robert K. Dornan, a California Republican, argued that HIV-infected troops constituted a threat to military readiness. He explained that because of the provision limiting the chronically ill to limited duty, they cannot serve overseas and must return to the United States during a time of cutbacks in defense resources. He added that the military could not afford to keep HIV-infected personnel if they were unable to perform all duties.

Responding to Dornan's plea to oust HIV-infected personnel, Frederick F. Y. Pang, the assistant defense secretary for force management policy, said discharging was unnecessary and would not improve military readiness. Pang wrote that if HIV-infected military personnel could perform required duties there was no reason to separate them from others or remove them from the armed forces. Dornan tried to pass a legislative provision (part of the proposed 1997 DOD authorization) that would discharge all HIV-positive military and would cut off benefits to dependents. But the House and Senate voted 399–25 to overturn the discharge law, which had been part of the 1996 DOD authorization.

Since 1985 the DOD has screened all new recruits, students entering the service academies, and those in the college Reserve Officers' Training Corps (ROTC) program. Those who test positive for HIV are not permitted into military service.

Pregnant Women and Newborns

The issue of testing newborns has placed the rights of mothers at odds with those of their newborns. States have kept HIV test results anonymous to preserve a mother's right to privacy. Civil libertarians and some groups that represent women, gays, and lesbians support anonymous testing, claiming that attaching names to test results would start local, state, and federal governments down the "slippery slope" of mandatory testing of adults. They also raise further privacy concerns, contending that once names are known, there is no guarantee they will not fall into the hands of employers, insurance companies, and others who might discriminate on the basis of HIV status.

On the other hand, proponents of disclosure claim newborns that test HIV-positive could be denied adequate medical care because their parents are unaware of their status. Approximately 75% of babies who test positive for HIV immediately after birth do not actually develop the disease. If their mothers breastfeed, however, the babies may contract the infection from their mother's milk.

In May 1996 the U.S. House and Senate passed bills that would cut off federal money for HIV/AIDS treatment to states that fail to comply with the new disclosure requirements. President Bill Clinton signed the Ryan White Comprehensive AIDS Resources Emergency (CARE) Act Amendment (PL 104–146) requiring mandatory testing of newborns if too few pregnant women agree to voluntary testing. States must now test all newborns for HIV and notify parents of the results. In June 1996 New York became the first state to mandate that health officials tell parents the results of HIV tests that the state routinely performs on all newborns. Before June 1996 parents in New York did not receive results unless they requested them, as was still the case in most states in 2005.

Health Care Workers and Patients

There has been a continuing debate over whether health care workers, who, many believe, have an obligation to inform their patients about their own HIV status, should be required to get tested. Some fear that mandatory testing of health care workers could eventually lead to mandatory testing of patients. In 1998 only patients who exhibited or claimed risk-taking behaviors or requested an HIV test were tested. In the medical setting in the early 2000s, however, all patients were treated as potentially infectious, and treatment personnel were required to wear protective gloves and, for some invasive medical procedures, goggles and masks. These safety measures are known as "universal precautions."

Prisoners

Screening prison inmates for HIV antibodies has been even more controversial than screening people in the general population. Prison officials feel pressure from lawmakers, city and county officials, correctional officers, and even some inmates to perform mandatory screening of all inmates and to make their HIV status known. Testing prisoners raises the issue of spending resources on screening instead of on educational materials to prevent infection. A number of prison systems engage in blind, anonymous prevalence studies where only overall results are made known and individual inmates are not told the test results. The majority of prison systems offer HIV testing for those who request it.

PREVENTION
Critics Fault Programs' Focus and Funding

The objective of HIV prevention programs is to reduce the number of new cases to as close to zero as possible. All prevention efforts are based on the belief that individuals can be educated in a way that will lead to changes in behavior, which will help bring an end to the spread of HIV/AIDS. But many AIDS advocacy groups have long been critical of the ways the CDC has communicated the message. In 1987 CDC officials decided to emphasize the universality of AIDS, instead of focusing its efforts on those most at risk—those who engage in male to male sexual activity (MTM) and intravenous drug users (IDUs). This strategy, according to AIDS advocates, misdirected the spending of available prevention dollars. Today, although the number of infected people outside of these two groups is growing, HIV/AIDS is still largely a threat to MTM, drug addicts, their partners, and their children. Most women with HIV/AIDS are drug users or sex partners of drug users.

This emphasis on the "anyone can get HIV" concept, critics claim, has diverted funds from the target populations with the greatest need for preventive health education. In 1995 the federal AIDS-prevention budget allocated no funds for programs aimed at MTM or for needle exchange programs. The CDC's 1996 $584 million AIDS prevention budget went largely to programs to help fight the disease among heterosexual women, college students, and others who face a relatively low risk of HIV infection. This policy continued into 2003.

CDC Prevention Activities

The CDC believes its role is to prevent HIV infection and to reduce the illnesses and deaths that result from HIV infection by working with communities and other partners. The agency's efforts focus on:

- Monitoring the epidemic

- Improving public understanding of the HIV epidemic

- Preventing risk behaviors among students

- Preventing and reducing behaviors and practices that transmit HIV

- Increasing individual knowledge of HIV status and improving referral to appropriate prevention and treatment services

According to the CDC, the most reliable ways to avoid HIV infection or transmitting the virus are abstaining from sexual intercourse, maintaining a mutually monogamous, long-term relationship with a partner who is uninfected, and/or to abstaining from sharing needles and/or syringes in drug use. While seemingly logical, critics contend that the emphasis of the CDC in particular, and of the administration of George W. Bush more generally, on abstinence burdens people with an unrealistic expectation. Critics also point to the insistence on abstinence policies as a condition in United States government assistance for other countries' health programs to be an ill-advised foreign policy intrusion.

The CDC's current HIV Prevention Strategic Plan has as its goal to "reduce the number of new HIV infections in the United States from an estimated 40,000 to 20,000 per year by the year 2005, focusing particularly on eliminating racial and ethnic disparities in new HIV infections." The CDC is devoting 10% of its AIDS budget to prevention efforts through FY 2005.

To accomplish their prevention goal, the CDC has adopted four specific criteria, which are to remain in effect beyond 2005:

- To decrease the number of people in the United States at high risk of acquiring or transmitting HIV by a minimum of 50%, by providing prevention interventions that are specific and ongoing, and that are based on evidence

- Increase the proportion of HIV-infected Americans who are aware of their HIV status from the current estimated 70% to 95%

- Increase the proportion of HIV-infected Americans who can get access to appropriate prevention, care, and treatment from an estimated 50% to 80%

- Increase the ability of national health agencies, including the CDC, to monitor the incidence and spread of HIV/AIDS, develop and initiate effective prevention strategies, and to evaluate the success of HIV/AIDS programs

The CDC's HIV prevention strategy has four components:

- To monitor the epidemic so that prevention and care activities can be strategically and appropriately targeted

- To research the effectiveness of the prevention methods

- To fund local prevention initiatives that target high-risk communities

- To develop fruitful linkages with care and treatment programs.

As part of this effort, the CDC stresses cooperation with, and provision of financial assistance and technical support to, state and local health and education agencies, national and local minority organizations, community-based organizations, schools and colleges, and business, labor, and religious organizations. The CDC distributes almost 75% of its HIV prevention funds through grants and contracts, primarily to state and local health and education agencies.

EDUCATING YOUTH

In 2001, 133,725 cases of AIDS in Americans between the ages of twenty and twenty-nine were reported to the CDC. With an average incubation period of ten years, it is likely that most of these young people were infected while they were teenagers. As some people begin having sexual relationships and using intravenous drugs at earlier ages, many fear the number of HIV-positive young people will grow.

Most states offer prevention programs for students in public schools. But youths who are not in school may not have ready access to such programs. Many homeless shelters and local health departments employ roving counselors who seek out these young people to offer prevention information and direct them to health and social service agencies.

Sexual Health Education

Many education programs offer students sufficient information about STDs and HIV/AIDS, but only high-quality education affects behavior. A 1997 review by the Joint United Nations Program on HIV/AIDS (UNAIDS) concluded that effective sexual education programs should include:

- Focused curricula, clear statements about behavioral goals, a clear picture of the risks of unprotected sex, and ways to avoid it

- Teaching and practice in communication and negotiation skills

- Openness in communicating about sex

- Theories stressing the social nature of learning

The review's conclusions have remained relevant and controversial. Even in 2005 some people do not agree that information about sexual decisions should be offered in public schools, preferring that parents instill their own values in their children. But others point out that some parents never talk to their children about sex and drugs, and school may be the only place a child can get reliable information. According to the National Conference of State Legislatures, forty states, the District of Columbia, Puerto Rico, and the Virgin Islands require HIV/AIDS prevention education. Though laws vary from state to state, and some allow local school districts to decide on curricula, many of these states have one or more man-

dates determining the material that may be taught in the programs. The mandates range from requiring age-appropriate materials, to teaching comprehensive sex education programs (advocating contraceptive and condom use), to providing programs in which abstinence from pre-marital sex is presented as the only 100% effective means of preventing HIV/AIDS.

Federal funding for abstinence-only educational programs, which was initiated in 1998, was cut in August of 2005. Proponents of these programs claim that they change attitudes about casual sex, reducing both teen pregnancies and rates of STDs. They also maintain that teaching students about contraceptive and condom use condones, or even encourages, unsafe sexual behavior. Critics of these programs argue that there is no reliable evidence that abstinence-only programs are effective. In addition, they contend that for the five out of ten teens ages fifteen to nineteen who do choose to have sex, lack of knowledge about contraception and condom use will only result in continued teen pregnancies, STDs, and HIV infections.

CONDOM USE

In June 2000 a workshop organized by the National Institutes of Health in collaboration with the CDC, the Food and Drug Administration, and the United States Agency for International Development evaluated published evidence on the effectiveness of latex male condoms in preventing STDs, including HIV. The results of the workshop were published in July 2001 (http://www.niaid.nih.gov/dmid/stds/condomreport.pdf). The publication stresses that studies provide compelling evidence that latex condoms are highly effective in protecting against HIV infection when used properly for every act of intercourse. But it warns that "no protective method is 100% effective, and condom use cannot guarantee absolute protection against any STD. Furthermore, condoms lubricated with spermicides are no more effective than other lubricated condoms in protecting against the transmission of HIV and other STDs."

While latex condom use is still considered a highly effective method of preventing the transmission of HIV and other STDs, the report concluded that abstinence or a mutually monogamous, long-term relationship with an uninfected partner is the "surest way to avoid transmission of sexually transmitted diseases."

Other Forms of Protection

In 1993 the FDA approved Reality, a female condom that serves as a mechanical barrier to viruses. The condom is designed for women to protect themselves from STDs, including HIV. It is made of polyurethane (a resin made of two different compounds used in elastic fibers, cushions, and various molded products) and is unlikely to rip or tear. The condom is prelubricated and is intended for use during only one sex act.

Spermicides, which contain the chemical nonoxynol-9 and are found in various lubricants used in conjunction with condoms in order to kill sperm and therefore further protect against pregnancy, were once thought to be a means of preventing HIV infection. As highlighted in the above-mentioned 2001 report, however, condoms lubricated with spermicides are no more likely to be effective than condoms used with other water-based lubricants.

IMPROVING PREVENTION SERVICES

In March 2000 community planners, health educators, and program directors met at the Community Planning Leadership Summit for HIV Prevention in Los Angeles, California, to share some of the most successful prevention and health education strategies from across the United States. By sharing these new and noteworthy "best practices," state health departments and local community planning groups were able to learn useful and proven approaches they could incorporate into their own programs.

The CDC reviewed the HIV prevention programs and compiled descriptions of them in a publication called *Bright Ideas 2000*. The publication was so well received that another edition, *Bright Ideas 2001: Innovative or Promising Practices in HIV Prevention and HIV Prevention Community Planning*, followed, profiling additional programs from several jurisdictions that had not been represented in the previous edition.

The latest edition available as of 2005, *Bright Ideas 2001*, describes programs that use innovative approaches to reach their target audiences, from an Alabama program that trained high school students to serve as peer group facilitators and counselors to an Iowa strategy to get members to arrive on time for meetings—latecomers were required to sing a song, tell a joke, or dance for the assembled group. A Louisiana program sought to improve its organizational ability to set priorities by using coded maps of STD rates, and in Maine a Web site helped people gain online access to HIV prevention information.

In 2000 the CDC also published the results of a study conducted by its Program Evaluation Research Branch (PERB), which tried to determine which factors help or hinder the efforts of community-based organizations (CBOs) that serve people at risk of acquiring or transmitting HIV. Using one-on-one and group interviews, PERB looked at twenty-six CBOs that varied in terms of target audience, geographic location, and type of services offered.

The PERB study found that some characteristics of the community—such as support from city and local health departments; well-organized target populations; strong, supportive families and faith organizations; and well-established social networks—were associated with the success of the CBOs in reaching their target audiences. Characteristics of the CBOs themselves that helped them to reach their target groups included a long history in the community; a strong, clear mission and identity; and a charismatic leader (one easily able to gain the trust and devotion of the group). Effective CBOs also established realistic goals and objectives, developed programs to meet clients "where they are at," and delivered information in an entertaining way. (See Table 8.2.)

Factors that hampered the effectiveness of the CBOs were high rates of poverty, racism, sexism, drug use, homophobia, teen pregnancy, and domestic violence, along with transient client populations. Policies that prevented condom distribution, not enough money to pay CBO staff, and limitations on the accessibility of syringes also prevented CBOs from reaching their target populations. (See Table 8.2.)

SYRINGE EXCHANGE PROGRAMS

Intravenous drug users (IDUs) often share the syringes they use to inject drugs into their body. If an HIV-positive IDU uses a syringe he or she may contaminate it with HIV-positive blood that can then cause the disease in other IDUs who use that syringe. Needle or syringe exchange programs attempt to prevent the spread of HIV in this manner by encouraging IDUs to bring in their used, unsafe syringes and exchange them for new, safe syringes. The reasoning behind these programs is that if people are going to use drugs, at least an effort can be made to make sure they do not contract HIV because of it. Proponents of these programs point out that the spread of HIV among IDUs threatens everyone, as people who contract HIV through drug use can then pass it on to their sexual partners and through childbirth. Federal officials estimate that each day thirty-three people are infected with HIV as a result of IDU. This figure includes IDUs, their sexual partners, and their children.

Despite these arguments, syringe exchange programs are highly controversial because of their connection to drug use. Some see them as helping IDUs avoid the consequences of their actions, or even providing them with the means to continue their illegal activities. In April 1998, after much debate, the Clinton administration decided not to lift a nine-year-old ban on federal financing for programs to distribute clean needles to drug addicts. This means that state and local governments that receive federal block grants for HIV/AIDS prevention are not permitted to use that money for needle exchange programs. Public health experts and advocates for people with HIV/AIDS criticized the decision. Later in 1998 Congress considered

TABLE 8.2

Factors that help and hinder community-based organizations in reaching their target populations and delivering interventions

	Factors that help	Factors that hinder
Structural/external	Supportive city and health department Well organized target population	Police harassment Limitations on the accessability of syringes Policies that prevent condom distribution Poverty Racism, sexism, drug phobia, homophobia
Cultural norms	Strong role of families Active faith communities	Distrust of social service providers Ashamed to talk about sexuality
Client factors	Well established social networks	High rates of drug use, poverty, unemployment, mental health issues, STDs, teen pregnancy, domestic violence, etc. Transient nature of clients Denial/clients tired of hearing about AIDS
Organizational	Long history in the community Credibility Clear mission/strong identity "One stop shopping": multi-services	Overly bureaucratic management Insufficient support for line staff Insufficient infrastructure Abstinence/no condom distribution policy
Staff	Charismatic leader Flexible work environment Support for line staff Staff represent community Commitment/work as a team	High turnover/vacancies Difficulty finding staff that represent target population Conflicts between staff Not enough money to pay staff
Program	Needs assessments Market research Realistic goals and objectives Incentives Meet clients "where they are at" "Infotainment"—combining education and entertainment Flexible implementation design	Unrealistic goals and objectives Inappropriate strategies for target population No meaningful integration of evaluation data

SOURCE: "Table 2. Examples of Factors That Help and Hinder CBOs to Reach Their Target Populations and Deliver Interventions," in *Learning from the Community: What Community-Based Organizations Say about Factors That Affect HIV Prevention Program*, Centers for Disease Control and Prevention, September 2000

even more restrictive legislation that would ban indirect federal funding (such as funding for counseling, medical care, or funds dispersed by city or state) to needle exchange agencies. Regardless, in 2000 five U.S. health groups (including the AMA and the American Pharmaceutical Association) spoke out in favor of needle exchange programs and advised state leaders to coordinate efforts to make clean needles easily available to IDUs.

The article "Update: Syringe Exchange Programs—United States, 1998" (*Monthly Morbidity and Mortality Report*, vol. 47, no. 31, August 14, 1998) summarizes a survey of U.S. syringe exchange program (SEP) activities during 1998. As of 2005 an updated survey has yet to be published. The survey was conducted in October 1999 by the Beth Israel Medical Center (BIMC) in New York City, together with the North American Syringe Exchange Network (NASEN). They mailed questionnaires to the directors of 131 SEPs in the United States who were members of NASEN. (Previous surveys contacted sixty-eight SEPs during 1994–1995, 101 in 1996, and 113 in 1997.) The BIMC contacted SEP directors and conducted telephone interviews based on the questionnaires. The directors responded to questions about the number of syringes exchanged during 1998, program operations, and services provided.

Of the 131 SEPs, 110 (84%) participated in the survey, but some asked that their data be reported only when considered along with all the data (aggregate reporting), rather than considering each jurisdiction separately. SEPs operated in eighty-one cities in thirty-one states, the District of Columbia, and Puerto Rico. The greatest numbers of SEPs were located in four states: California (21), New York (14), Washington (12), and New Mexico (9). Nine cities had at least two SEPs.

In 1998 the 107 individually reporting SEPs exchanged approximately 19.4 million syringes, up from the 1997 total of 17.5 million. The twelve largest SEPs (those that traded five hundred thousand or more syringes) exchanged approximately 12.1 million (62% of all replaced syringes). (See Table 8.3.)

In addition to exchanged syringes, most SEPs provided other public health and social services. Virtually all offered instruction in preventing sexual transmission of HIV and other STDs; 98% provided male condoms and 73% distributed female condoms. Ninety-nine percent provided IDUs with alcohol pads, 90% offered bleach to use as a disinfectant, and 95% referred clients to substance abuse treatment programs. Other on-site health care services provided by some SEPs included HIV counseling

TABLE 8.3

Syringe exchange statistics, 1998

Size	No. syringes exchanged per SEP	No. SEPs	Total no. syringes exchanged	% syringes exchanged
Small	<10,000	30	108,136	1%
Medium	10,000–55,000	26	778,701	4%
Large	55,001–499,999	39	6,398,409	33%
Very large	>500,000	12	12,112,281	62%
Total		**107**	**19,397,527**	**100%**

Note: SEP means syringe exchange program.

SOURCE: "Table 1. Number of Syringe Exchange Programs (SEPs), Number of Syringes Exchanged per SEP, Total Number of Syringes, and Percentage of Total Number of Syringes, by Program Size Category—United States, 1998," in "Update, Syringe Exchange Programs—United States, 1998," in *Morbidity and Mortality Weekly Report*, vol. 50, no. 19, May 18, 2001

and testing (64%), tuberculosis skin testing (15%), STD screening (14%), and primary health care (19%).

Helping IDUs Saves Lives

In "Changing Syringe Laws Is Part of Strategy to Help Stem HIV Spread" (*HIV/AIDS Prevention*, December 1997), the CDC points out that drug users must have access to clean syringes and drug treatment as part of a complete HIV prevention plan. One way to make this happen is to change the drug paraphernalia laws so that clean needles and syringes are available to IDUs. However, many people believe that by doing so the state is allowing drug use to take place, or even worse, condoning it.

The U.S. Public Health Service recommends that IDUs be counseled and encouraged to stop using intravenous drugs, if possible, through substance abuse treatment that includes relapse prevention. Failing this, however, drug users should follow various preventive plans that include:

• Never reusing or sharing syringes, water, or drug preparation equipment

• Using only syringes obtained from a reliable source (e.g., pharmacies)

• Using a new, sterile syringe to prepare and inject drugs

• Safely disposing of syringes after one use

Despite social and economic obstacles to their success, SEPs have repeatedly demonstrated that they can help change the lives of IDUs. Research reported in "A Drug Abuse Treatment Success among Needle Exchange Participants" (*Public Health Reports*, supplement 1, June 1998) found that 50% of clients referred for substance abuse treatment entered treatment and 76% completed thirteen weeks of treatment. These findings were especially impressive in view of the programs' clientele: people with more severe drug abuse, more HIV risk behaviors, and more participation in illegal activities than IDUs referred to treatment from other sites.

Legislation in Maine and Minnesota

A 1997 law in Maine (Maine Statute, Title 32, Ch. 117, Sect. 32, Para. 13787-A) permits anyone to legally possess ten or fewer syringes. "Illegal possession" of syringes applies to anyone who knowingly owns or furnishes eleven or more syringes, except those who must self-inject prescription drugs (like insulin-dependent diabetics) and SEP operators, who are not limited in the quantity of syringes they possess. The statute authorizes the state Bureau of Health to establish SEPs and set the rules that will govern them. SEPs must keep track of and dispose of syringes, they must have drug prevention education, and they are required to submit an annual report on the operation of their programs.

Legislation in Minnesota (Minnesota Statute Section 151 Para. 40) modified its drug paraphernalia law so that pharmacists are permitted to sell, and IDUs to buy, ten or fewer syringes. The state's commissioner of health is now required to give pharmacists help with technical issues, such as proper disposal of used syringes and provision of materials needed to make the program work.

Legal Barriers to Federal Funding of Needle Exchange Programs

Regardless of the evidence from a number of sources that needle exchange programs are effective strategies for the prevention of HIV transmission, the federal government, as well as most local and state governments, have not made them legal. They argue that illicit drug use should not be financed by taxpayers. Since 1988 Congress has passed at least six laws that contain provisions specifically prohibiting or restricting use of federal funds for needle exchange programs and activities. The Comprehensive Alcohol Abuse, Drug Abuse, and Mental Health Amendments Act of 1988 (PL 100–690) requires states, as a condition for receiving block grant funds, to agree that funds would not be used "to carry out any programs of distributing sterile needles for hypodermic injection of an illegal drug or distributing bleach for the purpose of cleansing needles for such hypodermic injection."

CHAPTER 9
HIV AND AIDS WORLDWIDE

SCOPE OF THE PROBLEM

Few factors have changed global demographics as inalterably as the pandemic (worldwide epidemic) of HIV/AIDS. As an illustration of this statement, United Nations (UN) officials projected that sub-Saharan African countries would be 4% less populated in 2005 than they would have been without the losses attributable to AIDS. Whether this prediction bears out awaits the publication of the United Nations–World Health Organization 2005 AIDS update. According to information released in 1996 by the International Programs Center of the U.S. Census Bureau, by 2025 the sub-Saharan population would have reached almost 1.3 billion without AIDS. A moderate spread of AIDS, however, could reduce that number by more than one hundred million.

The HIV/AIDS pandemic is actually many separate epidemics, each with its own distinctive origin and shaped by specific geography and populations. Each epidemic involves different risk behaviors and practices, such as unprotected sex with multiple partners or sharing intravenous drug equipment. According to the UNAIDS 2004 AIDS update, in a half-dozen sub-Saharan African countries the majority of the high-risk urban population—prostitutes and their customers and sexually transmitted disease (STD) patients—are HIV-positive. International authorities project that unless the rate of HIV/AIDS infection slows in thirteen sub-Saharan countries, Brazil, and Haiti, childhood mortality rates could triple by 2010.

In 1997 approximately 30.6 million people were infected with HIV, and the pandemic was growing by sixteen thousand new infections per day. By the end of 2004 the Joint UN Program on HIV/AIDS (UNAIDS) and the World Health Organization (WHO) estimated in "AIDS Epidemic Update: December 2004; Maps" (Joint United Nations Program on HIV/AIDS, http://www.unaids.org/wad2004/EPI_1204_pdf_en/Chapter11_maps_en.pdf,

December 2004) that approximately thirty-nine million people worldwide were living with HIV. This count included 17.6 million women and 2.2 million children younger than fifteen years. The report estimated that more than 13,500 new infections occurred each day, translating to almost five million new infections per year—4.3 million adults and 640,000 children in 2004. More than 95% of these HIV cases occurred in the developing world, particularly in sub-Saharan Africa and Southern and Southeast Asia. This number will increase as infection rates continue to rise in the face of poverty and inadequate health resources and health care infrastructure.

UN medical experts note that, before 1997, data coming from just a few countries in any particular area were used as models for other countries with comparable or fairly similar regional factors. As a result, for some countries the spread of HIV/AIDS was woefully underestimated. Beginning in 1997 separate models constructed for each country replaced regional models, resulting in more accurate statistics and projections.

UNAIDS estimated in AIDS Epidemic Update: December 2004; Maps (Joint United Nations Program on HIV/AIDS, http://www.unaids.org/wad2004/EPI_1204_pdf_en/Chapter11_maps_en.pdf, December 2004) that, in 2004, 3.1 million people worldwide died from AIDS, a marked increase from the 2.3 million deaths that occurred in 1997. Of these deaths, 2.6 million were adults and more than five hundred thousand were children younger than fifteen.

The 2004 UNAIDS report once again confirmed that the developing world bears the brunt of the AIDS misery. Approximately 64% of the world's HIV-infected population (25.4 million cases) lives in sub-Saharan Africa, while 18% (7.1 million cases) resides in South and Southeast Asia. Taken together, these two regions represent 82% of the world's HIV/AIDS population.

AIDS is also making inroads elsewhere. Until recently, AIDS in China had been largely confined to the traditional high-risk populations such as intravenous drug users (IDUs). But by 2002 the spread of the epidemic to heterosexual populations was clear. In Guangxi Province, for example, HIV infection rates among sex workers increased from 0% in 1996 to 11% in 2000. Another example is the Russian Federation and Eastern Europe, where HIV is increasing faster than anywhere else. In Ukraine nearly 25% of new infections occur through heterosexual encounters.

In order to understand the enormity and consequences of the AIDS pandemic worldwide, the focus should not be on the number of reported AIDS cases, but instead on the number of people infected with HIV (the virus that causes AIDS), most of whom have not yet developed full-blown AIDS. The HIV incubation period (the interval between the initial HIV infection and the development of AIDS) is estimated to be about seven to eleven years. With an estimated 4.9 million people newly infected in 2004 alone, the number of future AIDS cases will continue to increase dramatically.

Global Trends and Projections

Although public health programs have made impressive progress in eliminating and controlling many infectious diseases, HIV/AIDS is not one of them, according to the WHO. This is due to the constantly changing character and the complex role of factors that determine the progression from HIV infection to full-blown AIDS. In addition, medical treatments that can slow the progression of HIV are generally too expensive, and as a result inaccessible, for most people living in developing countries.

The World Bank projects that by 2020 AIDS will account for a large portion of deaths from infectious diseases in the developing world. In Latin America and the Caribbean, 74% of adults who die from an infectious disease will likely die from HIV/AIDS, while in the Middle East and North Africa only 18% of adults who die from an infectious disease will likely die from HIV/AIDS.

In 1990 HIV/AIDS accounted for 9% of adult deaths due to infectious diseases worldwide; but by 2020 HIV/AIDS is projected to account for 37% of adult deaths due to infectious diseases. The following observations describe the nature of the HIV/AIDS pandemic in 1998, which, without effective interventions, should develop in a similar manner through at least 2010:

- Most new HIV infections occurred in fifteen- to twenty-four-year-olds.

- Three-fourths or more (75 to 85%) of HIV-positive adults worldwide were infected through unprotected sex. Heterosexual intercourse accounted for more than 70%, and male to male sexual activity (MTM) accounted for 5 to 10%.

- Transfusions of HIV-infected blood caused 3 to 5% of all global adult infections.

- Sharing of HIV-infected injection equipment by drug users accounted for 5 to 10% worldwide.

- More than 90% of HIV-positive children throughout the world were infected by their mothers perinatally (before or during birth) or through breastfeeding. Approximately 30% of mother-to-child transmission took place through breast-feeding.

In the absence of expanded prevention and treatment efforts, the future outlook could be grim. UNAIDS projects that sixty-eight million people will die of AIDS by 2020, a toll that is more than five times the thirteen million deaths of the prior two decades in the developing world. Of the six million people in the developing world who are in need of HIV therapy (such as antiretroviral drugs), only 230,000 people were receiving such treatment at the end of 2001. "Access to adequate care and treatment is a right, not a privilege," Peter Piot, the executive director of UNAIDS, remarked in a press release announcing the publication of the 2004 UNAIDS AIDS update. Piot also remarked that although progress has been made, more action is needed to make sure that the people who need treatment get it. Costs must fall, and continued health care funding will be necessary.

Effect of AIDS on Death Rates

Life expectancy at birth is an important measure for comparing death rates within and between countries over time. In some countries hardest hit by AIDS, the number of years one may expect to live has returned to the levels of the 1960s. Other countries now have levels equivalent to those of the early 1990s, and child survival rates are slipping as well. Even in countries with a somewhat lower prevalence of HIV infection, AIDS accounts for 80% of deaths of people between twenty-five and thirty-four years of age, according to the UNAIDS report.

In the sub-Saharan African nation of Zimbabwe, one of the countries hardest hit by the AIDS pandemic, life expectancy is only forty-two years—twenty-two years less than it would be if not for the impact of AIDS. In Harare, the capital of Zimbabwe, deaths among children five years and younger rose from eight per one thousand population in 1988 to twenty per one thousand in 1996. In East Africa, where 10% of the rural population has HIV, adult mortality has more than doubled. In southern Africa life expectancy between 2005 and 2010 is expected to drop to forty-five years (from fifty-nine years in the early 1990s), largely as a result of AIDS. In the South American country of Brazil, one may expect a life span of sixty-two years, five years shorter than a decade ago. In the Asian country of Thailand, where strong prevention programs are in place, the life span is sixty-nine years, just two years shorter than a decade ago.

Because HIV/AIDS epidemics differ considerably from country to country, most current mortality estimates, especially in developing countries, do not accurately reflect the impact of AIDS-related mortality. The HIV/AIDS epidemic is changing the course of demographic events in developing countries where the impact has been particularly severe.

PATTERNS OF INFECTION

Globally, HIV/AIDS is primarily an STD, transmitted through unprotected sexual intercourse between men and women or MTM. Like some other STDs, HIV infection can also be spread through blood, blood products, donated organs, or semen, and perinatally from a woman to her unborn child. More than 75% of worldwide cumulative (over the entire time that statistics have been kept) HIV infections in adults are estimated to have been transmitted through heterosexual intercourse, although the relative proportion of infections resulting from heterosexual contact as opposed to MTM varies greatly in different parts of the world.

HIV-1 and HIV-2

Two types of HIV have been recognized and identified: HIV-1, the predominant worldwide virus, and HIV-2. HIV-1 and HIV-2 show an extraordinary difference in global distribution. In North and South America HIV-1 has reached epidemic proportions among certain risk groups, primarily through unprotected MTM contact and intravenous drug use. Some African and Asian countries have also experienced extensive heterosexual transmission of HIV-1. HIV-2 has spread among heterosexual populations in West Africa.

DIFFERENCES IN EPIDEMIOLOGY, INCIDENCE, AND TRANSMISSION. The epidemiological characteristics (factors such as distribution and incidence that determine the presence, extent, or absence of a disease) of HIV-2 are different from those of HIV-1. Perhaps reflecting these differences, the international spread of HIV-2 is quite limited. In the early course of infection, people with HIV-2 are less infectious than those with HIV-1. This is due to the low levels of the virus isolated from the blood of immunodeficient people with HIV-2. As time passes and an individual's immunodeficiency progresses, HIV-2 probably becomes more infectious, but this more infectious period is relatively shorter than for HIV-1 and tends to occur in older individuals.

Several studies provide reasonable evidence that HIV-2 is not frequently transmitted from mother to child. While the mechanics of perinatal transmission are not completely understood, advanced immunodeficiency of the mother is certainly a risk factor. Low levels of the virus are not sufficient to transmit to the baby and, as mentioned earlier, higher levels of virus infection in women past childbearing years may explain why perinatal transmission is less frequent. This is the most likely explanation for the observation that HIV-2 infection is so rare in children.

Compared to HIV-1, relatively little is known about how HIV-2 is spread. This may reflect the rarity of HIV-2 in the Western world, particularly the United States.

Interactions and HIV Transmission

One of the major concerns of public health officials worldwide is the possible interaction between HIV and other infections. The same risky behaviors that expose individuals to potential HIV infection also expose them to other STDs such as gonorrhea, syphilis, and chancroid (a genital ulcer). Considerable data suggests that STDs, particularly herpes simplex, chancroid, and syphilis (which all cause ulcerative lesions), promote the transmission of HIV.

TUBERCULOSIS. HIV infection is recognized as the strongest known risk factor for the development of active tuberculosis (TB), since people with latent TB infection are more apt to develop the disease once their immune system has been compromised by HIV. Latent TB infection is believed to be present in about 30 to 50% of adults in most developing countries. People with latent TB have positive tuberculosis skin tests but are not sick with tuberculosis—they have been infected with *Mycobacterium tuberculosis* at some point in their lives but have not developed active TB.

Up to 8% of people infected with both latent TB and HIV are expected to develop active TB each year. The WHO estimates that at least four million adults worldwide, primarily in sub-Saharan Africa, Latin America, and Asia, have been infected with both HIV and *M. tuberculosis*. Not only are people infected with HIV who test tuberculin-positive more likely to develop TB, they are also likely to develop TB more rapidly than people without HIV infection. An even more disastrous consequence is that half of all people infected with both will develop contagious TB, which they could then spread to any susceptible individual, even those not infected with HIV. Currently, TB kills about two million people annually in developing countries, a figure that has grown dramatically since the HIV/AIDS epidemic has swept through many countries. The number of cases will continue to grow.

Geographic Differences

In North America and Western Europe during the 1980s and early 1990s, HIV was transmitted predominantly through unprotected sexual intercourse among MTMs and through intravenous drug use (IDU) with contaminated needles. During the late 1990s heterosexual intercourse and IDU became the prevailing modes of HIV transmission in North America and Europe.

In sub-Saharan Africa the overwhelming mode of transmission has been heterosexual intercourse. In that part of the world, transmission through MTM contact or through IDU is slight. Because many women have been infected, rates of perinatal transmission are increasing. In 2004, 90% of HIV-positive babies born worldwide were in sub-Saharan Africa.

The rates of MTM transmission in Latin America are similar to those of Europe and the United States, but IDU is less frequent, while heterosexual transmission is considerably higher. In South and Southeast Asia, the rapid increase of HIV can be traced to shared contaminated injection equipment and heterosexual intercourse.

In other areas, such as East Asia and the Pacific region, the predominant modes of transmission are not as clearly defined because of the relatively recent (late 1980s) spread of HIV in these areas. While the infection rate has peaked in other parts of the world, it is escalating in Asia, mainly from heterosexual intercourse through prostitution. According to UNAIDS, in 2003 South and Southeast Asia had between 700,000 and 1.3 million adults and children living with HIV, representing an average of 1.0 million. By the end of 2004 the estimated numbers were 4.4 to 10.6 million, representing an average of 7.1 million and a sevenfold increase over the previous year.

AFRICA

Rural Africa Catching Up

Studies conducted in remote areas of the African country of Zaire in both 1976 and 1985 revealed HIV in only about 1% of the hundreds of people tested. At the time HIV was a rarity and existed at a stable level. In urban areas, however, the virus spread through increased sexual activity and the relaxation of traditional tribal values. As more poor rural workers left their villages to search for jobs, the epidemic spread. Able-bodied workers often could not (and still cannot) bring their families with them when they leave their homes to seek work, and many took new sexual partners in the cities where they worked. These workers returned to their villages, bringing HIV and other STDs with them.

Unparalleled Infection Rates

In early 1997 the South African government estimated that 2.4 million South Africans were living with HIV. UNAIDS estimated that by the end of 2004 25.4 million adults and children in sub-Saharan Africa were infected. The national prevalence rates (the number of cases of the disease present in a specified population at a given time) of HIV infection among adults varied widely. Some West African countries report less than 2%. Others, in the southern portion of the continent, experience much higher rates. For example, in Botswana—which has the highest HIV infection rate in the world—almost 39% of adults were living with HIV at the end of 2001, an increase from 36% only two years before. In Zimbabwe—where 25% of adults were HIV-positive in 1997—one-third of the adult population was infected with HIV at the end of 2001.

SEVERAL MODES OF TRANSMISSION. Because heterosexual transmission is the predominant mode of transmission in Africa, men and women appear to be almost equally infected (twelve to thirteen females per every ten males). Commercial sex workers, or prostitutes, and their customers play a significant role in the spread of HIV in many countries. In many African cities the risk of contracting HIV infection approaches 50%. In some cities infection is rampant, especially among sex workers in the lower classes.

In the late 1990s four out of five HIV-positive women in the world lived in Africa, as did 87% of children who lived with HIV. There are several reasons for this. The female childbearing population is larger in Africa than any other place, and African women generally have more children than women in other parts of the world. This means that one woman can pass the virus on to more children. Furthermore, nearly all children in Africa are breastfed, and breastfeeding is responsible for more than one-third of mother-to-child transmissions of HIV. Although there are new drugs and drug combinations available to sharply reduce mother-to-child transmission, they are expensive and women in developing countries generally cannot afford them.

In response to routine screening of donated blood and the more careful use of blood for procedures such as transfusions, the role of transmission through HIV-infected blood has diminished considerably over the past several years, accounting for less than 10% of the total reported HIV infections. Ancient practices of ritual scarification and the use of improperly sterilized skin-piercing instruments (such as needles and syringes) account for a very small proportion of all HIV infections in sub-Saharan Africa.

PAYING THE PRICE FOR YEARS OF EVASION. Although their country had experienced the ravages of AIDS for about a decade, Kenya's Parliament and cabinet did not debate the issue publicly until 1993. Physicians diagnosed the first AIDS cases in 1984, but the government did not issue national statistics until 1986, when it announced one AIDS-related death. Although the nation's president and vice president regularly warned the public in speeches to avoid infection, and national officials instructed district administrators, including local tribal chiefs, to encourage their people to practice safe sex and limit their partners, there had been no official statement.

The government's belated commitment to dealing with HIV/AIDS came too late for many Kenyans. By 2000, 2.1 million citizens had been infected with HIV, representing nearly 15% of all sexually active adults. About six hundred deaths per day in Kenya are attributable to AIDS, and by 2005 this number is projected to climb to 820 deaths per day (as of mid-2005 the projection was unconfirmed). Moreover, the National AIDS/STD Control Program (NASCP) estimates that more than 730,000 Kenyan children under the age of fifteen have lost their mothers to AIDS. NASCP projects that this number will reach one million by 2005 (unconfirmed as of mid-2005).

The Kenyan government's reticence and seeming inability to deal with the epidemic came as a surprise to many observers. Kenya has endured an economic decline that many blame on corruption and the collapse of global commodity prices. Nonetheless, Kenya is still one of Africa's wealthiest countries and has remained relatively stable since gaining its independence from Britain in 1963. Many observers thought that if any African country could cope with or even head off an HIV/AIDS epidemic, it would be Kenya.

But Kenyan officials chose to downplay the threat, lest it frighten away much-needed tourist dollars. By contrast, Kenya's neighbor Uganda began an aggressive campaign against the spread of HIV/AIDS in the mid-1980s, when it had the highest number of recorded HIV cases in Africa. With virtually every family touched by HIV/AIDS, much of the cultural, religious, and psychological stigma has disappeared in Uganda, where HIV infection rates now appear to be declining. In Kenya, on the other hand, many HIV-infected people still mistakenly believed, many years after the epidemic first hit, that the absence of symptoms meant they were not infected.

Faced with an epidemic that by 2010 will orphan more than 30% of Kenyan children under age fifteen, Kenyan authorities have now developed a long-term strategy to deal with HIV. In 1997 Parliament adopted Sessional Paper No. 4. The law called for a vigorous campaign aimed at changing society's attitudes toward casual sex and proposed that anyone who intentionally infects another with HIV be found guilty of manslaughter.

Much of the HIV/AIDS epidemic in Kenya and other nations of East Africa can be attributed to the preponderance of wars and political upheaval. In addition, many prostitutes reside along long-haul truck routes linking Tanzanian and Kenyan ports to land-locked interior nations: Ethiopia, Uganda, Rwanda, Burundi, and the eastern part of Zaire. Male and female adolescents between the ages of fifteen and nineteen have begun to frequent truck stops along the Trans-Africa Highway in Kenya. Teenagers in families that cannot adequately provide them with food and clothing trade sex for money and gifts.

International experts report that HIV in these areas is also prevalent among people with higher-paying jobs, such as businessmen in Nairobi and Mombasa and truck drivers who frequent the roads between the eastern coast and the interior. It is not uncommon or socially unacceptable for a man of means to have a family as well as a couple of girlfriends. As in other parts of Africa, the big cities draw men from rural areas in search of work. Separated from their families for several months, many of these men turn to prostitutes and eventually contract HIV and carry it home to their villages. A considerable number of women in the cities who are abandoned or need additional income turn to prostitution to eke out a living.

"Wife inheritance" was once a socially useful tradition; now it is a large contributor to the ever-increasing spread of HIV/AIDS. In western Kenya, when a woman is widowed, her former husband's family takes care of her and her children. For generations, a brother-in-law or male cousin took her in with his family. Initially, tradition frowned on his having sexual relations with the inherited wife. Unfortunately, the inheritors began to ignore that restriction and had sex with the widow. If the widow's former husband had died of AIDS, she was likely to be infected and could pass the infection on to her inheritor, who would pass it on to his wife, causing the disease to multiply exponentially.

UGANDA'S DECLINING HIV RATES. Scientists think that more than twenty years ago truck drivers first spread HIV in Uganda's Rakai District, which lies along a Lake Victoria trade route to the capital city of Kampala. Because commercial sex is widely available along the trade route, HIV quickly spread throughout Uganda and all of Africa. At one time, Uganda had the world's highest HIV infection rates. By the early 2000s it became one of only two developing nations (Thailand is the other) where there was nationwide evidence of declining HIV rates due to strong prevention programs. According to the UN, Uganda reduced the prevalence of HIV infection by more than one-third, from almost 13% in 1994 to 8% in 1998.

Uganda was the first African country to respond strongly to its HIV/AIDS epidemic. The government began by gathering religious and traditional leaders, along with representatives of other sectors of society, in an effort to reach agreement that the problem had to be confronted. Prevention efforts targeted specific populations or communities. For example, prevention programs that focused on delaying sex and behaving in a safe manner were presented in schools. Community groups were formed to counsel and support those living with the virus. Condom use was heavily promoted.

Infection rates, particularly for the young, have begun to fall in both rural and urban surveillance sites. In 1989, according to the UN, 69% of fifteen- to nineteen-year-old males and 74% of fifteen- to nineteen-year-old females reported that they had had sexual intercourse. By 1995 those percentages had dropped to 44% among the young men and 54% among the young women. Young Ugandans seem to be postponing sexual initiation, seeking fewer sexual partners, and using condoms more.

EUROPE

Western Europe

While HIV in Europe is spread primarily through MTM contact, intravenous drug use is gaining as a mode of transmission. In the mid-1980s about 63% of AIDS cases among adult Europeans was due to MTM contact; by the early 1990s that proportion had dropped to 42%. Meanwhile, the proportion of European AIDS cases attributable to IDU jumped more than sevenfold, from 5% in the mid-1980s to 36% in the early 1990s, where it has remained through 2005.

According to the Centers for Disease Control and Prevention (CDC), the reported number of AIDS cases stabilized in 1994 and 1995. In 1996 the number of AIDS cases reported throughout the European Union (EU) dropped about 10%. In 1997 CDC statistics indicated that the AIDS epidemic had declined sharply in Western Europe (39%); UNAIDS reported thirty thousand new cases in Western Europe that same year. Since the late 1990s the decline appears to have leveled off; just over thirty thousand new cases were reported in 2002, and 570,000 people were estimated to be living with HIV/AIDS at the end of that year. The majority of HIV transmissions in Spain and Italy was through IDU, while in France, Germany, and the United Kingdom, it was through MTM contact. Mother-to-child transmission rates were low due to the availability of antiretroviral drugs for pregnant women and safe alternatives to breast-feeding for HIV-infected mothers. UNAIDS estimated that fewer than five hundred children under the age of fifteen were infected with HIV in 2002.

SPAIN. Spain has the highest number of HIV/AIDS cases per capita in the European Union. The first case of HIV was reported in Spain in 1981; by the end of 2001, 110,000 to 150,000 people were living with HIV. In 2001 alone 2,500 to 3,000 new cases were reported. Spain accounts for one-fourth of all HIV cases in Western Europe. (Italy and Portugal also have high rates.)

Drug use in Spain began to increase during the 1970s and 1980s after the long Franco dictatorship ended. Isabel Noguer of the Health Ministry describes this period as a time of heavy heroin use, with addicts sharing infected needles. In 1997 drug users still made up the highest risk group, while unprotected heterosexual relations was the next most common form of transmission. According to Spain's Health Ministry in 2000, 56% of HIV infections among men and 48% among women were attributable to intravenous drug use, while heterosexual transmission was responsible for 22% of all cases (male and female).

Spain developed education and prevention programs, and the number of new cases began to level off in 1996. The Health Ministry gives more than $1 million in aid to two hundred nongovernmental groups annually. Condom sales in the mid-1990s were double the number in the 1980s. These efforts appear to have been effective. The number of AIDS cases dropped 13% from 1999 to 2000, and from 1995 to 2000 there was an overall decrease of 64% in reported AIDS cases and an 85% reduction in cases of mother-to-infant transmission of HIV.

Eastern Europe

The HIV epidemic did not reach Eastern Europe until the mid-1990s. According to the UN, only 31,000 out of 450 million people were infected in 1995 throughout all of Eastern Europe. By 1997 about 190,000 adults were infected with HIV, and by the end of 2002 an estimated one million people throughout Eastern Europe were infected. By the end of 2004 the figure was estimated at 1.4 million people. Intravenous drug use has been the primary source for the spread of the virus.

Ukraine and the Russian Federation have been the hardest-hit countries in Eastern Europe, showing the steepest increase in HIV infection from 1996 to 1999. According to estimates by UNAIDS and the WHO, the former Soviet Union, as well as the rest of central and Eastern Europe, saw a one-third increase in the total number of HIV infections during 1999. In the entire east European region during 1998 and 1999, 90% of AIDS cases reported during that period were from Ukraine. As of 2004 HIV continued to spread at a rapid pace in the Russian Federation.

In 1994 only forty-four people in Ukraine tested positive for HIV. In 1996 more than twelve thousand tested positive, and in 1997 fifteen thousand more new infections were identified. In 2000 an estimated 250,000 people were living with HIV/AIDS in Ukraine. The story is much the same in the Russian Federation. In 1994, 165 people tested positive for HIV; most of those cases were attributed to MTM contact, while only two of the cases were reported among IDUs. In 1997 nearly forty-four hundred people tested positive, three times as many as in 1996. In 1998 four out of five newly diagnosed cases were reported IDUs. During 2000 nearly sixty thousand new cases of HIV infection were reported, far more than the twenty-nine thousand cases registered in the twelve years between 1987 and 1999. The proportions of the epidemic may be significantly underestimated since, by its own admission, the Russian system manages to register only a small proportion of all cases.

ASIA

Asia—home to two-thirds of the world's population—could eventually overtake Africa as the continent most affected by HIV. The HIV/AIDS epidemic arrived in Asia much later than in the rest of the world. Until the mid-1990s HIV/AIDS was uncommon, but because the average incubation period is approximately ten years, more people are now beginning to die from the disease. UNAIDS estimates that the number of Asian adults and children infected with HIV exceeded eight million at the end of 2004, with an estimated 1.2 million Asians contracting the infection that year alone.

Most countries in Southeast Asia have been hard hit, with the exception of Indonesia, Laos, the Philippines, and Sri Lanka. In these countries fewer than one out of one thousand adults was infected in 1999. Most of the Southeast Asian countries have not developed sophisticated systems for monitoring the spread of HIV, so estimates are often made using less information than in other regions of the world. In populous countries small differences in reported rates can mean a large difference in the actual numbers of infected people.

Thailand

The spread of HIV in Thailand had been almost unprecedented. Thailand's commercial sex industry is notorious, and travel packages based on the availability of sex workers in Thailand are common in Asia (as they are in other countries, including the United States). In the capital city of Bangkok, brothels are found in virtually every neighborhood. A 1990 survey found that 20% of all Thai men reported they had paid for sex in the previous year. After a military coup in 1991, the transitional government instituted a comprehensive AIDS education program, which included a media campaign and condom distribution to brothels and massage parlors. Brothels that refused to use condoms were closed down. While the anti-HIV program came too late for those infected in the mid- to late 1980s, Thailand recorded a drop in new HIV infections until the late 1990s.

Unfortunately, HIV appears to be spreading among other high-risk groups, such as IDUs and MTM, who have not received as much attention in prevention campaigns. According to UNAIDS, in 2001 an estimated 2% of adult males and 1% of adult females in Thailand were living with HIV/AIDS. The majority of those 675,000

adults are believed to be sex workers, their clients, and IDUs. Even if effective prevention measures continue, the epidemic will claim fifty thousand Thais every year until 2006. The HIV infection rate is expected to persist in excess of 1.5% among adult males. In addition, more than 90% of AIDS deaths will occur in people ages twenty to forty-four, the mainstay of the workforce.

Other Southeast Asian Countries

In other parts of Southeast Asia, current statistics on the epidemic show different patterns. As mentioned earlier, Indonesia, Laos, the Philippines, and Sri Lanka still record low rates of HIV infection. The reasons for the low rates are not clear. Moreover, there are no guarantees that prevalence will remain low. Some early indicators suggest changing patterns of incidence and prevalence.

Cambodia is the hardest-hit country in the region, with an estimated prevalence of 2.8% infected in 2000. According to a 2001 survey published by the Cambodian National Center for HIV/AIDS, Dermatology and STD (NCHADS), one out of thirty pregnant women, one out of sixteen soldiers and police officers, and one out of every two sex workers tested positive for HIV. Condom use has become much more common, with sales rising from zero to one million units per month in fewer than three years. But commercial sex is still very popular. In a recent survey three-fourths of respondents in the military and the police force and two-fifths of male students reported visiting a prostitute in the previous year.

In Myanmar (formerly Burma) HIV infection among sex workers rose from 4% in 1992 to more than 20% in 1996, and nearly two-thirds of IDUs are infected. Tests of pregnant women in six urban areas showed that approximately 2% were infected with the virus. UNAIDS estimates the prevalence at about five hundred thousand HIV/AIDS cases in 2000 and projects the addition of as many as fifty-five thousand adult cases per year by 2005 (a projection that remains unconfirmed in mid-2005, pending publication of the UNAIDS 2005 annual global AIDS survey).

India

At the International AIDS Conference held in Vancouver, British Columbia, in July 1996 a UN official reported that India had emerged as the country with the most people infected with HIV. This news came as a surprise to many of the conferees because HIV was not detected in India until 1986. In fact, by the end of 1993 only five thousand AIDS cases had been reported to the WHO from all of Asia. In 2000, according to the UNAIDS program, about five million of India's 950 million people were HIV-positive. Little is known, however, about how the infection flourished so quickly.

Although surveillance is irregular, recent testing indicates that the virus continues to spread. In Pondicherry, in the southeastern area of India, about 4% of pregnant women have tested positive. The states of Maharashtra, Tamil Nadu, Karnataka, Andhra Pradesh, and Manipur reported prevalence rates higher than 1%. AIDS deaths were estimated at 350,000 in 2000 and about a half a million are anticipated in 2005.

In March 1996 industrialists in India launched a nationwide campaign to educate their workers about HIV and help prevent its spread. Most of India's HIV-infected population resides in the cities, especially Mumbai (formerly Bombay), the country's financial capital, and along trade routes lined with brothels that serve truck drivers. Mirroring the situation in some regions of Africa, the infection rate among Indian prostitutes is upward of 50%. With India's population of one billion people, half of whom are illiterate, the task of instituting effective HIV education and prevention programs is a daunting one for the government.

China

The first HIV case in China was identified in 1985, but the disease did not begin to spread until the early 1990s, when changes in the structure of the economy produced an increase in drug use and prostitution. At the end of 1996 the government of China estimated that as many as 250,000 people were living with HIV/AIDS, approximately 10% of them teenagers. By the beginning of 1998 that estimate had doubled. By 1999 half a million Chinese were estimated to be HIV positive, and by the end of 2000 the estimate had risen to six hundred thousand. As noted earlier, by the end of 2002 indications were that HIV was spreading throughout China, affecting mainly heterosexuals. Despite these estimates, the confirmed cases were much lower. By March 1998 only 9,970 HIV infections were confirmed, up from 8,277 in September 1997.

The HIV/AIDS epidemic appears to be growing largely among two groups in China. One is among IDUs in the southwestern portion of the country; the other, newer epidemic is among heterosexuals along the eastern seaboard. Prostitution along the eastern coast of China is growing as the gap between rich and poor widens. The number of reported cases of STDs has escalated sharply in recent years, a sure warning sign of the high-risk behavior that leads to HIV/AIDS. Paid blood donations are on the rise as well, and this is also fueling the rapid spread of the virus through donated blood that is contaminated.

In 1997 the UN gave China a $1.8 million grant to help fight the disease over a four-year period. The funds were used to train ministry workers and to increase prevention education among high-risk populations. Although HIV education programs are common in urban areas, they have not reached the rural areas, where, when questioned, one-third of medical workers could not explain how HIV was transmitted.

Estimates of Chinese AIDS deaths in 2004 ranged from sixty thousand to one hundred thousand. Most of these likely occurred in the provinces where HIV prevalence is already high: Yunnan, Xinjiang, Guangxi, and Sichuan.

Overall, through 2004 about 8.6 million people were believed to be living with HIV in Asia and the Pacific—about 22% of the world's total cases, according to the UN. The huge populations of India and China dominate any assessment of HIV. Because the countries have so many inhabitants, small percentage changes in the estimates of national infection rates result in large changes in the estimates of the total number of people infected. For example, a rise of just 0.1% prevalence among adults in India would add more than a half million people to the national total of adults living with HIV.

LATIN AMERICA

According to UNAIDS, through 2004 an estimated 1.7 million adults and children in Latin America were living with HIV. An estimated 240,000 adults and children became infected that year.

Initially, the majority of HIV/AIDS cases in Latin America could be traced to MTM transmission. However, as of 2004, the greatest increases were among IDUs, although there were also increases attributable to heterosexual transmission. Levels of transmission among MTM in urban areas of Brazil, Mexico, Argentina, and Honduras range from 20 to 35%. There are also indications of high HIV infection rates among commercial sex workers in some areas. As a rule, infection rates among IDUs have reached or exceeded 30%. In Brazil HIV infection rates among IDUs have been reported to be as high as 40% in Rio de Janeiro, 54% in Sao Paulo, and 57% in Santos.

The picture in Latin America is mixed. In some countries prevalence is rising rapidly, but in other parts of Latin America infection rates are falling or remaining stable. Nearly every country in Latin America now reports HIV infections. More than half report concentrated epidemics. These include the most heavily populated countries in the region: Brazil and Mexico.

The spread of HIV in Latin America mirrors the pattern of that in industrialized countries. MTM and IDUs who share needles continue to make up the highest risk groups. Studies done in Mexico indicate that about 14% of MTMs may be living with HIV. Between 3 and 11% of IDUs in Mexico are infected. In Argentina and Brazil the proportion may be closer to half.

Rates are rising for women, which is indicative of an increase in the heterosexual transmission of the virus. In 1986 one out of seventeen AIDS cases in Brazil were in women. By 1997 the number was one out of four—one-fourth of the 550,000 adults living with HIV in Brazil were women. In Latin America and the Caribbean during 2000 about 210,000 adults and children became HIV infected, and an estimated 1.8 million were believed to be living with HIV/AIDS. About one-fifth of those infected were women. By the end of 2002 UNAIDS estimated that 1.9 million people were living with HIV/AIDS in Latin America and the Caribbean. By the end of 2004 that figure had increased to an estimated 2.1 million.

Several Latin American countries are beginning to establish programs to help care for those living with HIV/AIDS, including programs that provide life-prolonging antiretroviral drugs. For example, in Brazil more than eighty-five thousand people with HIV received government-subsidized antiretroviral therapy during 2000. Although overall access to care is better in Latin America than in most other areas of the developing world, it is not consistent throughout the region.

THE CARIBBEAN

In 1982 the first suspected AIDS cases in the Caribbean appeared in Jamaica. Since then, the epidemic has changed from a mostly homosexual phenomenon to a heterosexual one, with 65% of reported cases resulting from heterosexual transmission, according to UNAIDS. About 35% of all HIV-infected adults in the Caribbean are women, and the prevalence rate among pregnant women has been rising each year. Unlike in other parts of the world, in the Caribbean the connection between HIV and intravenous drug use is low. But the rapidly growing popularity of crack cocaine and the traditionally common practice of men (and, more recently, women) having multiple sexual partners are fueling the spread of HIV.

Through 2004, an estimated 440,000 adults and children in the Caribbean were living with HIV, and fifty-three thousand had contracted the infection during that year, according to UNAIDS.

Caribbean countries are confronting an epidemic that has left the region with the world's second-highest incidence rate after sub-Saharan Africa. According to UNAIDS, in 2000 Haiti was the Caribbean nation hardest hit; about 8% of adults in urban areas and 4% in rural areas were infected, as were 13% of pregnant women who were anonymously tested. According to UNICEF (http://www.unicef.org/infobycountry/index.html), 2001 prevalence rates among adults were 3.2% in Trinidad and Tobago and 1.7% in the Dominican Republic. UNAIDS estimates that at the end of 2004, 440,000 people were living with HIV/AIDS in the Caribbean.

A number of factors contribute to these high prevalence rates:

- For many years, some Caribbean governments did not want to admit the problem for fear of losing their tourist trade.

- The area has seen years of political and social unrest.

- There are high poverty rates and low levels of education.

- Many Caribbean communities are vulnerable because of their socioeconomic disadvantages and lack of information.

- Migration among countries and from rural to urban areas contributes to the continued spread of HIV and makes it harder to prevent.

- There is little tolerance for MTM in the Caribbean, which means that many governments were unwilling to fight the disease until recently, when officials realized that most HIV/AIDS patients in the Caribbean were heterosexuals.

THE MIDDLE EAST AND NORTH AFRICA

Less is known about HIV infection rates in North Africa and the Middle East than in other regions of the world. According to UNAIDS, through 2004 an estimated 540,000 adults and children were infected with HIV, with ninety-two thousand acquiring the infection during that year.

Middle Eastern countries with large numbers of immigrant workers carry out mass screenings for the virus, but no estimate places the number of infections at more than one adult in one hundred. The infection rate is estimated to be a low 0.13%. Approximately 220,000 adults and children are thought to be living with HIV in these countries. In Djibouti and Sudan, an estimated 2.9 and 2.3%, respectively, of those between the ages of fifteen and forty-nine were infected with HIV at the end of 2003, according to statistics from UNICEF. These were markedly higher than the other reporting Middle Eastern countries.

Because social and political attitudes in the Middle East and North Africa are generally conservative, it has proven difficult for governments to deal with risky behavior directly. Nonetheless, there are some community and nongovernmental organizations that help sex workers and IDUs whose behaviors put them at risk for HIV infection.

The WHO reports that in Middle Eastern countries HIV/AIDS is viewed as a social stigma associated with MTM, a practice strongly disapproved of by the cultures and religions of the region. A large number of North African and Middle Eastern countries cannot be classified because of lack of data. Although limited data is available, there are indications that extensive spread of HIV has begun in some parts of the region, with 18% of adult deaths from infectious disease resulting from HIV/AIDS. The epidemic in the Middle East was just beginning in 1998, but there is some evidence that HIV infections are increasing among IDUs in Bahrain and Egypt. Although drug use is also frowned upon in these conservative cultures, trade in addictive drugs such as heroin appears to be substantial in some parts of the region.

CONTROVERSIES

While great strides have been made in treating HIV infection and AIDS, and in raising public awareness about the nature of the disease and preventing its spread, several controversies dampen the enthusiasm about the fight against AIDS being effective worldwide.

Prohibitive Cost of Treatment in Developing Countries

A study conducted by the Rand Corporation and published in the *New England Journal of Medicine* in 2001 estimated that in 1998 treatment of HIV in the United States cost about $1,410 per month, or nearly $17,000 for the year. The additional treatment costs for AIDS can inflate the annual tally to more than $70,000. Even in a wealthy country like the United States, this is beyond the reach of most Americans. In the developing world, where the annual income can be only several hundred dollars, this treatment cost can prove absolutely prohibitive in the absence of government subsidies for HIV treatment.

Government subsidies can provide relief. A study published in the July 15, 2005, issue of *Clinical Infectious Diseases* reported that countries like Botswana that have government-funded AIDS treatment programs to provide free or low-cost treatment achieve greater treatment success than countries that do not provide such subsidized assistance. In the case of Botswana, six months after the initiation of the subsidized program, almost 30% more patients had undetectable viral levels when they received the drugs at no cost than did those who had to pay.

However, as the study's authors pointed out, this success could only be maintained in the long term if the drugs are either provided free of charge to the countries through an international aid program or can be obtained at a substantially lower cost than was the case as of 2005.

Cost of Treatment

The high price of HIV/AIDS drugs is a contentious issue. While manufacturers did freeze their prices briefly in 2002, they subsequently began to raise them again. In February 2003, for example, Roche announced that the price of Fuzeon, then the most expensive AIDS treatment on the market, would more than double in Europe.

As with other drugs, some advocate for the availability of generic versions of HIV/AIDS treatment drugs. Generic drugs invariably carry a lower purchase price than their patent-protected counterparts. But without the benefit of the market exclusivity that patent protection carries for the company that develops a drug, the motivation to continue the search for new drugs might vanish. A pharmaceutical manufacturer must cover the cost not only of research and development for the approximately three out of ten drugs that succeed, but also for many of the drugs—seven out of ten—that fail to make it to the marketplace. Because of this cost, once a new drug receives Food and Drug Administration (FDA) approval its manufacturer typically has the exclusive right to market the drug, usually for anywhere from three to twenty years. This allows the manufacturer to recoup its investment and realize a profit. During this time the drug is priced much higher than if other manufacturers were allowed to compete by producing generic versions of the same drug. The lower cost of the generic versions reflects the fact that the generic manufacturer does not have to pay for the successes and failures that occurred in the drug development pathway or pursue the complicated, time-consuming process of seeking FDA approval. The producer of generic drugs has the formula and must simply manufacture the drugs properly. Because of the lower cost of the generic drug after the original patent or exclusivity period has expired, competition among pharmaceutical manufacturers generally lowers the price. HIV/AIDS drugs are granted seven years of exclusivity under legislation aimed at encouraging research and promoting development of new treatments.

The concern over patent protection for HIV/AIDS drugs is understandably contentious. In contrast to generic versions of, for example, cold medications, HIV/AIDS drugs can literally be lifesavers. Pharmaceutical manufacturers argue that patent protection is vital to alleviate the financial burden associated with drug development. However, to those directly affected by HIV/AIDS, and those governments or health care systems that provide care, especially in developing countries, the enormous costs can be infuriating, especially with the knowledge that generic drugs carrying a lower price tag are possible.

In November 2002 the World Trade Organization (WTO) adopted a resolution affirming that the governments of WTO member countries have the right to take whatever actions they deem necessary to protect public health, including overriding pharmaceutical patents. In May 2003 the government of Zimbabwe declared a national emergency for six months over the HIV/AIDS pandemic, enabling it to purchase and make available generic versions of HIV/AIDS drugs that are still under patent protection. Prior to this, the passage of the Kenya

Industrial Property Bill 2001 allowed the importation and production of more affordable medicines for HIV/AIDS in that country.

Tying Foreign Policy Aid to Abstinence

Another controversial issue surrounding HIV/AIDS treatment is the U.S. foreign policy initiative in place in 2005—dubbed the President's Emergency Plan for AIDS Relief (PEPFAR)—that ties funding for developing countries to programs that stress abstinence as the only prevention option.

Abstaining from sexual intercourse does prevent the sexual transmission of HIV, although most experts, who agree that it is not realistic to expect sexual abstinence from many segments of the population, stress that condom use is essential in stopping the spread of the disease. Reflecting President George W. Bush's 2004 State of the Union Address, which urged a new emphasis on abstinence-only education and doubled the funding for abstinence-only programs, abstinence is a critical part of PEPFAR. Launched in 2003, PEPFAR is a five-year, $15 billion program intended to fight the spread of HIV/AIDS in twelve African countries and the Caribbean. South Africa received almost $90 million in PEPFAR funds in fiscal year 2004 and is expected to receive another $149 million between October 2005 and September 2006. A third of PEPFAR's money goes to programs promoting sexual abstinence, and prevention efforts that focus on the promotion of monogamy (having just one sex partner) are favored.

Many AIDS activists decry PEPFAR, saying it slights the Global Fund to Fight AIDS, Tuberculosis and Malaria, set up in 2002. The United States has committed only $200 million a year to the Fund, far short of the expected contribution. Many critics also believe that PEPFAR attempts to export the Bush administration's conservative ideology globally.

In mid-2005 the United States Agency for International Development (USAID) cut funding to Population Services International (PSI)—a Washington, D.C.-based nonprofit group that promotes healthy behavior and products to low-income people in seventy developing countries—because Republican senator Tom Coburn of Oklahoma voiced his objections to a PSI program in Central America that used easy-to-understand games to encourage illiterate prostitutes to use condoms to prevent the spread of HIV/AIDS. According to Helene Cooper, writing in the *New York Times* ("What? Condoms Can Prevent AIDS? No Way!," August 26, 2005, http://www.nytimes.com/2005/08/26/opinion/26fri4.html?n=Top%2fOpinion%2fEditorials%20and%20Op%2dEd%2fEditorials), Coburn wrote to President Bush that the PSI program was a "misuse of funds to organize and sponsor parties and dance contests to exploit victims of the sex trade." PSI regional executive director Michael Holscher countered that the games were "a simple activity for largely illiterate people" to encourage and teach proper condom use among a high-risk population. PSI says of its Central American anti-AIDS programs, run by its regional affiliate, Pan-American Social Marketing Organization (PASMO): "As many as 57% of CSWs [commercial sex workers, or prostitutes] in some Central American countries benefited from PASMO activities, resulting in both a reduced number of occasional clients and reported high and consistent condom use with clients" ("Reaching Vulnerable Girls and Women through a Balanced and Targeted Approach," *PSI Profile*, August 2005, http://www.psi.org/resources/pubs/womenHIV.pdf). Several other members of the U.S. Congress raised their own objections to the funding cuts, urging USAID to restore the money to PSI's programs.

According to the Web site of the organization Human Rights Watch (http://hrw.org/campaigns/aids/2005/uganda/):

> "Abstinence-only" programs (like PEPFAR) teach that abstaining from sex until marriage is the only effective way to prevent contracting HIV through sex. They deny young people critical information about condoms and other safer sex strategies, and promote marriage as a safeguard against HIV infection. These programs do not work, they violate kids' right to complete information about HIV/AIDS and leave young people at risk of contracting HIV in marriage, particularly women and girls.

CHAPTER 10

KNOWLEDGE, BEHAVIOR, AND OPINION

CONCERNS ABOUT HIV/AIDS

By the early 2000s the American public appeared less concerned about HIV/AIDS and its impact on health care than ever before. According to Gallup polling, in 1988 more than two-thirds of all Americans named AIDS as the most urgent health problem facing the country. In 1993 41% identified AIDS as the most pressing problem, and another 30% named health care costs. But in 1997 29% of poll respondents cited AIDS as the most urgent health problem, 15% named cancer, and another 15% cited health care costs.

The 2000 Gallup Poll marked the first time since 1987 that AIDS did not top the list of Americans' health care concerns. AIDS was third, trailing health care costs and cancer. In 2000 just 18% of Americans considered AIDS the most urgent health problem. Among young Americans ages thirteen to seventeen, AIDS was rated the second most urgent health problem plaguing the country. Fourteen percent of young Americans cited AIDS, while 16% named cancer the number one problem. By October 2001 AIDS had dropped even lower on the list of Americans' concerns, as they focused on the more immediate issues of the economy and unemployment, terrorism, fear of war, and national security.

Over time people have grown less concerned about personally acquiring AIDS. According to *Gallup Poll Monthly*, in October 1997 30% expressed some concern about getting the disease, down from 42% who felt that way in 1987. A Henry J. Kaiser Family Foundation survey conducted by Princeton Research Associates from August 14 to October 26, 2000 (still the most current data as of mid-2005), explored the attitudes, beliefs, knowledge, and opinions about HIV/AIDS. Using data provided by the Roper Center for Public Opinion Research at the University of Connecticut, the survey of 2,683 adults found only 19% of respondents "very concerned"

about becoming HIV infected, and an additional 18% said they were "somewhat concerned." Thirty-nine percent of survey respondents reported that they were "not at all concerned" about becoming infected with HIV.

Some attitudes about HIV have not changed much. When asked if they were more or less concerned about a son or daughter becoming infected with HIV than they were a few years ago, 47% of respondents to the Kaiser Family Foundation survey said they were "about as concerned." A similar proportion (50%) reported that they were "about as concerned" that they themselves would become infected as they were a few years ago. The remainder was about evenly divided between feeling more concerned (22%) and less concerned (25%) about becoming infected.

KNOWLEDGE AND TOLERANCE GROW

During the more than two decades since the virus that is believed to cause AIDS was first identified, aggressive community health education and awareness programs have sought to increase the public's knowledge about HIV/AIDS. Based on the findings of the 2000 Kaiser Family Foundation survey, American adults are better informed than ever before about HIV/AIDS.

The majority of people surveyed (89%) know that there is no cure for AIDS; 88% know that there are no drugs available that cure HIV. Almost as many (79%) are aware that there is not yet a vaccine that protects against becoming infected with HIV.

In 1997 Americans were slightly more tolerant of those who contracted AIDS than they were in 1987. In 1987 43% believed that AIDS was a punishment for the decline in moral standards. In 1997 31% of those questioned felt that way. In 1997 40% of poll respondents said that people have themselves to blame if they get AIDS, down from 51% in 1987.

Further illustrating the decreasing social stigma of HIV infection, the Kaiser Family Foundation survey found that about two-thirds of respondents believed they would not be thought badly of if people found out they had been tested for HIV. Fifty-two percent said they would be "not at all concerned" that people would think less of them if it were discovered they had been tested for HIV. An additional 13% said they would not be too concerned if people found out they had been tested for HIV.

Beliefs about Preventing HIV/AIDS

One of the biggest changes in the way Americans view HIV/AIDS is reflected in the fears and misconceptions people have about catching the disease. In 1987 43% of those surveyed said that they avoided associating with people who might have HIV/AIDS; by 1997 the number had dropped to only 15%. While 28% of respondents in 1987 said that they did not use public rest rooms in order to lessen their chances of coming into contact with the virus, just 12% of those asked in 1997 agreed with the statement. And in 1997 33% of Americans polled said they would avoid elective surgery requiring blood transfusions due to concern over the blood supply in hospitals, compared with the 42% who felt that way in 1987. One of the most extreme measures of preventing the spread of HIV would be to isolate people with HIV/AIDS from the rest of society. Twenty-one percent of those polled in 1987 believed this proposal was a good idea; in 1997 only 7% did.

People who responded to the Kaiser Family Foundation survey expressed support for other measures to prevent the spread of HIV/AIDS. Fifty-eight percent favored needle exchange programs that offer clean needles to intravenous drug users (IDUs) in exchange for used needles, and 60% thought state and local governments should be permitted to use federal funds for needle exchange programs. A comparable proportion (61%) would allow IDUs to purchase clean needles from licensed pharmacists, and 60% said physicians should be able to offer IDUs prescriptions for clean needles.

Preventing the spread of HIV is important to the people surveyed. Nearly all believed that research to develop a vaccine to prevent HIV infection should be a priority of the federal government; 83% considered it very important; and 13% felt it a somewhat important government responsibility. The survey respondents were divided about the top priority for the federal government—44% favored vaccine research and 41% chose AIDS prevention and treatment.

TEEN ATTITUDES

American teens are worried about HIV/AIDS. Indeed, the majority of U.S. teens view HIV/AIDS as a serious problem for their generation. In 2000, 34% of those polled said they were very concerned about becoming infected. This finding is from the Kaiser Family Foundation's *National Survey of Teens on HIV/AIDS 2000*, which looks at attitudes and knowledge about HIV/AIDS in a representative sample of teens ages twelve to seventeen (as of 2005, the survey had not been repeated). The national survey also found that more African-American and Hispanic teens felt very concerned about becoming HIV infected than white teens. (See Figure 10.1.)

The overwhelming majority (more than 90%) of teens surveyed knew that sharing needles and having unprotected sex place them at risk of HIV infection. This may reflect the fact that more schools, churches, synagogues, youth groups, the media, and parents are teaching kids about HIV/AIDS and informing them about how the disease is spread. Still, not all teens are fully aware of the health behaviors that place them at risk; only 69% identified oral sex as a risk and just 41% knew that having another sexually transmitted disease (STD) increases the risk of HIV infection. (See Figure 10.2.)

Though they may be better informed because they have grown up with the HIV/AIDS epidemic, 48% of teens still wanted to know more about HIV/AIDS and how it is spread, while 55% wanted to know where to get tested for HIV. More than half (57%) of the teens surveyed wanted to learn how to protect themselves from HIV infection, and 46% wanted to know how to talk to a partner about HIV/AIDS. Slightly fewer teens (40%) wanted instruction about how to talk with their parents about HIV/AIDS, and 36% would like to learn the proper way to use condoms. (See Figure 10.3.)

African-American and Hispanic teens and teen girls of all races and ethnicities reported the highest levels of interest in learning more about HIV/AIDS. Although many teens have been touched by the epidemic—overall one in six said they knew someone who had tested positive for HIV, had AIDS, or died from AIDS—one in four African-American and Hispanic teens knew someone affected by HIV.

MISINFORMATION PERSISTS

In 1997 a random telephone poll of 1,712 adults reported at the 12th World AIDS Conference in Geneva, Switzerland, in July 1998 found that about half of American adults erroneously believe that drinking from the same glass as an HIV-positive person can transmit the virus. The study also found that about three-fourths of American adults think that immigrants, pregnant women, and others at risk should be routinely tested for HIV infection.

FIGURE 10.1

Teens' personal concern about becoming infected with HIV/AIDS, 1998 and 2000

Percent who are "very" or "somewhat" concerned, 1998 and 2000

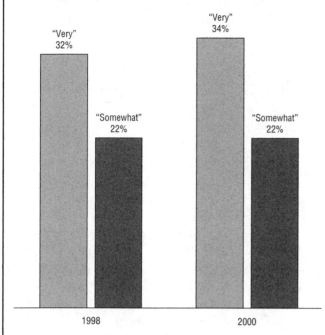

Percent who are "Very" concerned, by race/ethnicity, 2000

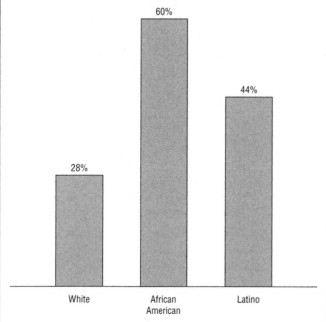

SOURCE: "Figure 1. Personal Concern about Becoming Infected," in *Kaiser Family Foundation National Survey of Teens on HIV/AIDS, 2000*, The Henry J. Kaiser Family Foundation, Washington, DC, 2000. Reprinted with permission of the Henry J. Kaiser Family Foundation of Menlo Park, California. The Kaiser Family Foundation is an independent health care philanthropy and is not associated with Kaiser Permanente or Kaiser Industries.

FIGURE 10.2

Teens' knowledge about risk of infection with HIV/AIDS, 2000

Percent of teens who are aware of the increased risk of infection for...

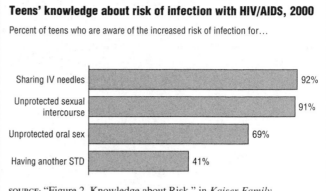

SOURCE: "Figure 2. Knowledge about Risk," in *Kaiser Family Foundation National Survey of Teens on HIV/AIDS, 2000*, The Henry J. Kaiser Family Foundation, Washington, DC, 2000. Reprinted with permission of the Henry J. Kaiser Family Foundation of Menlo Park, California. The Kaiser Family Foundation is an independent health care philanthropy and is not associated with Kaiser Permanente or Kaiser Industries.

FIGURE 10.3

Teens' desire for knowledge about HIV/AIDS, 2000

Percent of teens who want to know more about...

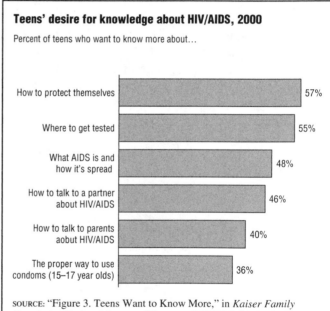

SOURCE: "Figure 3. Teens Want to Know More," in *Kaiser Family Foundation National Survey of Teens on HIV/AIDS, 2000*, The Henry J. Kaiser Family Foundation, Washington, DC, 2000. Reprinted with permission of the Henry J. Kaiser Family Foundation of Menlo Park, California. The Kaiser Family Foundation is an independent health care philanthropy and is not associated with Kaiser Permanente or Kaiser Industries.

In 2004 these erroneous beliefs concerning HIV transmission persist, despite massive public awareness campaigns by organizations including the Centers for Disease Control and Prevention (CDC) and the World Health Organization (WHO).

The World AIDS Conference research also indicated that, along with incorrect ideas about how the disease is spread, the stigma surrounding HIV/AIDS might be on the rise. Twenty-nine percent thought that anyone who contracted AIDS through drug use or sex had "gotten what they deserve," up from 20% of people in 1991. Twenty-five percent of respondents believed that people with AIDS are reckless and do not care about infecting others. The percentage of those who thought HIV could be spread by a shared drinking glass actually climbed from 48% in 1991 to 55% in 1997.

Fifteen years after the disease began to spread in the United States, it was still greatly misunderstood. More than one-fourth (27%) of those surveyed said they would be less likely to wear a sweater that had been worn once by a person with AIDS, even if the sweater had been cleaned and stored in a sealed package. One-third said they would not shop in a grocery store owned by someone who had AIDS.

Of course, one cannot generalize from the data of a single small study. But the figures serve as an interesting benchmark of our general societal views and indicate how little we have progressed in our understanding of HIV/AIDS and our compassion for those who are its victims.

One explanation offered for this persisting high level of misinformation is that most HIV/AIDS education is geared toward populations at high risk and not the general population. According to Wes Kennedy, the education coordinator for the AIDS Prevention Project at the University of Texas Southwestern Medical Center in Dallas, people who do not see themselves at risk may not be as receptive to public health education. But he agrees that the fact that so many people continue to believe old myths is frightening.

HISPANICS ARE MORE AFFECTED BY HIV/AIDS

In 2003 Hispanics made up about 13% of the U.S. population but accounted for 18% of all AIDS cases cumulatively diagnosed through that year, according to the CDC. Hispanic women are seven times more likely to become HIV infected than non-Hispanic whites, and almost one in four children under age thirteen diagnosed with AIDS is Hispanic.

In May 1998 the Kaiser Family Foundation conducted a nationwide telephone survey in Spanish and English. One-half of Hispanics surveyed believed AIDS was the United States' most serious health problem, and two-thirds said that HIV/AIDS was a serious problem for someone they knew. When compared to the overall adult population, nearly twice as many Hispanics said that they were "very worried" about becoming infected with HIV (24 and 46%, respectively).

According to the survey, most Hispanics (98%) knew that HIV/AIDS is a sexually transmitted disease, and 92% were aware that a pregnant woman could pass the infection on to her baby. But only 77% knew that there is no cure for AIDS, and even fewer (68%) were aware that there is no vaccine to prevent HIV.

Jane Delgado, the president of the National Coalition of Hispanic Health and Human Service Organizations, emphasizes that prevention strategies and education approaches must be tailored to address HIV/AIDS-related problems particular to individual communities. For example, most Hispanics living in the Northeast were infected with HIV through intravenous drug use, while male to male sexual activity (MTM) was the major cause of infection among Hispanics in Florida, California, and the Southwest. Delgado also expressed the view that there is a need to adapt education and prevention materials so that people from all backgrounds can understand them.

PEOPLE WITH HIV/AIDS

Behaviors chiefly associated with increased risk for sexual transmission of HIV by infected people include unprotected sex and intravenous drug use. But therapeutic regimens for HIV infections seem to be having a positive effect. Speaking at the annual meeting of the Infectious Disease Society in San Francisco in 2002, Daniel Kaswan of the Infectious Disease Clinic at Montefiore Medical Center in New York presented the findings of a survey he and other researchers conducted in 2001. The researchers interviewed eighty men and eighty women who were HIV infected and receiving treatment at the Infectious Disease Clinic. Even among the 60% of survey participants who had been diagnosed with AIDS, 70% said their health had improved over the past year. Two other findings also surprised the researchers: most patients (70%) could accurately predict the results of their laboratory tests and even those with full-blown AIDS rated their health as good.

FAILING TO INFORM A PARTNER

Between 1994 and 1996 researchers at Boston City Hospital and Rhode Island Hospital questioned 203 HIV-infected patients receiving treatment, 129 of whom reported sexual activity in the previous six months. Four out of ten HIV-infected people surveyed at these two New England hospitals failed to tell their sex partners about their condition, and nearly two-thirds of those did not always use a condom.

Those questioned were mostly poor intravenous drug users who did not have a high school education. People with only one sexual partner were three times more likely to have told their partner than those who reported multiple partners. Predictably, those with supportive partners were more likely to disclose their HIV infection. Whites and Hispanics were three times as likely to tell their partners as were African-Americans.

Of those who were sexually active, 46% were African-American, 27% were white, and 23% were Hispanic. Of those questioned, 41% were infected through intravenous drug use, 39% through heterosexual contact, and 20% through MTM contact.

Michael Stein, an associate director of the Brown University AIDS Program in Providence, Rhode Island, has noted that previous surveys of MTM produced similar findings, especially the greater likelihood that a person with one partner would admit HIV status than would a person with multiple partners. According to Stein, the problem is not one of knowledge, but of personal responsibility.

Failure to disclose HIV status or delaying telling a sex partner may be related to an HIV-infected person's social support system; those without close family, friends, and established sex partners may be less likely to reveal their HIV status. Researchers Lea Trujillo, Megan O'Brien, and their colleagues at Tulane University's School of Public Health and Tropical Medicine interviewed 269 people treated in New Orleans HIV clinics during the summer of 2000. Of the men and women surveyed, 52% were African-American and 80% reported becoming infected through heterosexual contact.

Nearly three-quarters of those with regular sex partners reported that they had disclosed their HIV infection to their partners, and 70% told their immediate families. In contrast, only one-quarter of people with casual sex partners said they had disclosed their HIV infection to their partners. Furthermore, those who did not tell their partners about their HIV infection were less likely to use condoms than those who had disclosed their HIV status to at least one casual sex partner.

Presenting the study at the October 2001 annual meeting of the American Public Health Association, O'Brien warned that people who look and feel healthy while taking antiretroviral drugs may mistakenly assume that this effective treatment is a cure. O'Brien encouraged health professionals to teach patients about the importance of disclosure and how to tell their sex partners about their HIV infection. She cautioned uninfected people that they "cannot assume partners will volunteer their HIV status" and reminded them that they must assume responsibility for practicing safe sex.

IMPORTANT NAMES AND ADDRESSES

AIDS Action
1906 Sunderland Place, NW
Washington, DC 20036
(202) 530-8030
FAX: (202) 530-8031
E-mail: aidsaction@aidsaction.org
URL: http://www.aidsaction.org

**American Foundation for AIDS Research
(amfAR)**
120 Wall Street
13th Floor
New York, NY 10005-3908
1-800-392-6327
(212) 806-1600
FAX: (212) 806-1601
URL: http://www.amfar.org

**Center for Women Policy Studies
National Resource Center on Women
and AIDS Policy**
1211 Connecticut Avenue, NW
Suite 312
Washington, DC 20036
(202) 872-1770
FAX: (202) 296-8962
E-mail: cwps@centerwomenpolicy.org
URL: http://www.centerwomenpolicy.org

**Centers for Disease Control and
Prevention (CDC)**
1600 Clifton Road
Atlanta, GA 30333
1-800-311-3435
(404) 639-3311
URL: http://www.cdc.gov

**Centers for Disease Control and
Prevention (CDC) National Prevention
Information Network**
P.O. Box 6003
Rockville, MD 20849-6003
1-800-458-5231
FAX: 1-888-282-7681
E-mail: info@cdcnpin.org
URL: http://www.cdcnpin.org/scripts/
index.asp

**Food and Drug Administration (FDA)
Center for Drug Evaluation and Research**
1451 Rockville Pike,
#6027
Rockville, MD 20852
(301) 594-6740
FAX: (301) 594-6197
URL: http://www.fda.gov/cder

Henry J. Kaiser Family Foundation
2400 Sand Hill Road
Menlo Park, CA 94025
(650) 854-9400
FAX: (650) 854-4800
URL: http://www.kaisernetwork.org

**House Energy and Commerce Committee
Subcommittee on Health and the
Environment**
2125 Rayburn House Office Bldg.
Washington, DC 20515
(202) 225-2927
URL: http://energycommerce.house.gov

Human Rights Campaign
1640 Rhode Island Avenue, NW
Washington, DC 20036-3278
(202) 628-4160
FAX: (202) 347-5323
E-mail: hrc@hrc.org
URL: http://www.hrc.org

National AIDS Fund
1030 15th Street, NW
Suite 860
Washington, DC 20005
1-888-234-AIDS
(202) 408-4848
FAX: (202) 408-1818
E-mail: info@aidsfund.org
URL: http://www.aidsfund.org/naf

National Association of People with AIDS
8401 Colesville Rd.
Suite 750
Silver Spring, MD 20910
(240) 247-0880

FAX: (240) 247-0574
E-mail: info@napwa.org
URL: http://www.napwa.org

**National Association of Public Hospitals
and Health Systems**
1301 Pennsylvania Avenue, NW
Suite 950
Washington, DC 20004
(202) 585-0100
FAX: (202) 585-0101
URL: http://www.naph.org

National Hemophilia Foundation
116 W. 32nd Street
11th Floor
New York, NY 10001
1-800-424-2634
(212) 328-3700
FAX: (212) 328-3777
E-mail: info@hemophilia.org
URL: http://www.hemophilia.org

**National Institute of Allergy and
Infectious Diseases (NIAID)**
31 Center Drive, MSC 2520
Bldg. 31, Room 7A50
Bethesda, MD 20892-2520
(301) 496-5717
FAX: (301) 402-0120
URL: http://www.niaid.nih.gov

National Minority AIDS Council
1931 13th Street, NW
Washington, DC 20009
(202) 483-6622
FAX: (202) 483-1135
E-mail: info@nmac.org
URL: http://www.nmac.org

National Women's Health Network
514 10th Street, NW
Suite 400
Washington, DC 20004
(202) 347-1140
FAX: (202) 347-1168
URL: http://www.womens
healthnetwork.org

The Orphan Project
121 Avenue of the Americas
6th Floor
New York, NY 10013
(212) 925-5290
FAX: (212) 925-5675
URL: http://www.aidsinfonyc.org/
orphan

UNAIDS
20 Avenue Appia
CH-1211 Geneva 27
Switzerland
(+4122) 791-3666
FAX: (+4122) 791-4187
E-mail: unaids@unaids.org
URL: http://www.unaids.org

U.S. Department of Health and Human Services AIDSinfo
P.O. Box 6303
Rockville, MD 20849-6303
1-800-448-0440
FAX: (301) 519-6616
E-mail: contactus@aidsinfo.nih.gov
URL: http://www.aidsinfo.nih.gov/live_help

RESOURCES

The Centers for Disease Control and Prevention (CDC) in Atlanta, Georgia, a division of the U.S. Public Health Service, in its *Morbidity and Mortality Weekly Report* (*MMWR*), offers the most current accounting of the HIV/AIDS epidemic. Articles used in this publication from *MMWR* include "Revised Surveillance Case Definition for HIV Infection, 1999" (vol. 48, no. RR-13, 1999); "Update: Syringe Exchange Programs—United States, 1998" (vol. 50, no. 19, 2001); and "Acquired Immunodeficiency Syndrome (AIDS). Number of reported cases, by year—United States and U.S. territories, 1983–2003."

The *HIV/AIDS Surveillance Reports*, prepared by the CDC, are published twice a year. The reports include details of transmission categories, risk factor combinations, demographics, people living with HIV, and the number of health care professionals who tested positive for HIV and AIDS through December 1997. Other CDC publications used to prepare this publication include *The 1993 Expanded AIDS Surveillance Case Definition* (1993) and *The 1994 Revised Classification System for Human Immunodeficiency Virus Infection in Children Less Than 13 Years of Age* (1994).

The National Center for Health Statistics (NCHS) in Hyattsville, Maryland, a division of the U.S. Public Health Service, publishes the findings from the *National Health Interview Survey in Advance Data*. *Survey* findings include "National Ambulatory Medical Care Survey: 2000 Summary" (2000). The NCHS also provides an overall picture of the nation's health in its annual publication *Health, United States, 2002*.

The Department of Justice, in its Bureau of Justice Statistics *Bulletin: HIV in Prisons and Jails, 2002*, provides information on HIV/AIDS in America's prisons and jails, inmate deaths from HIV/AIDS, and testing policies for the virus antibody by states.

Information on funding appropriated through the Ryan White Comprehensive AIDS Resources Emergency (CARE) Act was published in *Ryan White CARE Act of 1990—Opportunities to Enhance Funding Equity* (Washington, DC, 1995) and *HIV/AIDS—Use of Ryan White CARE Act and Other Assistance Grant Funds* (Washington, DC, 2001, 2002, 2003, 2004) by the Government Accountability Office. The Health Resource and Services Administration Division of the U.S. Department of Health and Human Resources provided recent information on funding for the CARE Act.

Information about the worldwide effects of HIV/AIDS, as well as projections for 2004 and beyond, were provided by reports from the World Health Organization and the United Nations Program on HIV/AIDS, both located in Geneva, Switzerland. The American Association for World Health (Washington, DC) also provides information and current facts on HIV/AIDS around the world and in the United States.

The Henry J. Kaiser Family Foundation publishes the results of surveys conducted by Princeton Research Associates using data provided by the Roper Center for Public Opinion Research at the University of Connecticut. The publication *Kaiser Family Foundation National Survey of Teens on HIV/AIDS, 2000* was used to prepare this publication. The Kaiser Family Foundation also provides daily updates about a variety of issues related to HIV/AIDS at its online site, http://www.kaiser-network.org.

Information about many facets of HIV/AIDS may be found at the online site http://www.thebody.com. Several articles from the site were used in this publication. The online sites http://www.biospace.com and http://www.homedrug-test.com provided information about HIV home testing options. The status of pediatric AIDS is also covered in this publication, using information in part from the Elizabeth Glaser Pediatric AIDS Foundation. The online Housing and Urban Development site (http://www.hud.gov) provided information on housing opportunities for people with HIV/AIDS.

Figures from *Confronting AIDS: Public Priorities in a Global Epidemic* (New York: Oxford University Press, 1997) and from *1998 World Development Indicators* (Washington, DC, 1998) by the World Bank were helpful. In addition, figures and information from *AIDS Epidemic Update: December 2002* (Washington, DC) were published by the World Health Organization and the United Nations Program on HIV/AIDS.

The Gallup Organization, Inc., publisher of the Gallup Polls, supplies timely data about public attitudes and opinions. We appreciate the Massachusetts Medical Society's tables from the *New England Journal of Medicine* article "Physician-Assisted Suicide and Patients with Human Immunodeficiency Virus Disease" (Lee R. Slome et al., February 6, 1997). The Pharmaceutical Research and Manufacturers of America published the figure displaying pharmaceutical research and development spending in *PhRMA Annual Survey, 2002*.

INDEX

CD4+ T cells
HIV/AIDS case definition and, 13, 14
HIV/AIDS progression and, 8
Celebrities, with HIV/AIDS, 79–81
Centers for Disease Control and Prevention (CDC)
adolescents and HIV/AIDS, 56
AIDS among heterosexuals and, 39
AIDS definition by, 13
AIDS infection, clinical categories of, 15t
AIDS rates among MTM, 28
children with HIV infection, statistics on, 52–54
classification system for HIV infection, expanded surveillance case definition for AIDS among adolescents and adults, 14t
condom use workshop, 92
estimate of people living with HIV/AIDS, 1
health care provider guidelines, 64–65
hemophiliacs and AIDS, 46
HIV/AIDS in Europe, 102
HIV/AIDS prevention activities, 91–92
HIV testing and, 89
HIV transmission in health care setting, 65–66
home testing and, 89
life expectancy of children with HIV, 54–55
mortality from AIDS, 36–37
1993 Revised Classification for HIV Infection and Expanded AIDS Surveillance Case Definition for Adolescents and Adults, 13–14
number of people infected with HIV, 23
on office visits, 61–62
older people with HIV/AIDS, 81
pediatric HIV classification, 50–51, 50 (t5.1)
prevention services, 93
resources on HIV/AIDS, 117
revised surveillance case definition, 2000, 14–15
safety of blood/transplant procedures, 19, 20
study on dementia and AIDS, 16
syringe exchange programs, 94–95
women and AIDS, 42
"Centers of Excellence" program, 61
Cervical cancer, 13–14
Cesarean section (C-section), 42, 51
"Changing Syringe Laws Is Part of Strategy to Help Stem HIV Spread" (Centers for Disease Control and Prevention), 95
Children
AIDS cases by race/ethnicity, 34
children < 13 years of age living with HIV infection or AIDS, estimated rates for, 29f

diagnosis of HIV infection in children, 50 (t5.2)
estimated numbers of persons living with HIV infection or AIDS, by state or area of residence, age category, 24t–25t
HIV/AIDS case definition for, 50–51
HIV/AIDS in, 49–50
HIV/AIDS in Africa, 100
HIV/AIDS in Europe, 102
HIV/AIDS in Latin America, 104
HIV-positive mothers having babies, 54
in Kenya, 101
mortality from AIDS, 37
number living with HIV/AIDS, 23
number of AIDS cases, 30
number of HIV-infected children, 52–54
pediatric HIV classification, 50 (t5.1)
perinatal infection, 51–52
reported cases of HIV infection, by age category, transmission category, sex, 53t
survival of/problems of, 54–55
treatments for, 52
worldwide infection patterns, 99
worldwide number with HIV/AIDS, 97
worldwide perinatal infection of, 98
Children's Evaluation and Rehabilitation Center of the Albert Einstein College of Medicine, 55
Chimpanzee, 4–5
China
HIV/AIDS in, 98, 104
HIV quick-response tests in, 22
HIV urine tests in, 21
Chinese National Center for AIDS Prevention and Control (NCAIDS), 21
Cigarettes, 9
Clinical Infectious Diseases, 106
Clinton, Bill
CARE Act and, 90
Medicaid coverage for HIV-infected people, 59–60
syringe exchange program and, 93
Clotting factor, 46
Coburn, Tom, 107
Community-based organizations (CBOs), 93, 94t
Community Planning Leadership Summit, 93
Comprehensive Alcohol Abuse, Drug Abuse, and Mental Health Amendments Act of 1988, 95
Concerns, about HIV/AIDS, 109
Condoms
abstinence programs and, 107
HIV/AIDS in Asia and, 103
partner notification and, 112, 113
Population Services International and, 107
to prevent STDs, 56

for prevention of HIV transmission, 75
in Uganda, 102
Conference on Retroviruses and Opportunistic Infections, 10
Confidentiality
contact tracing/partner notification and, 89
name-based reporting and, 87–89
Confronting AIDS: Public Priorities in a Global Epidemic (World Bank), 118
Connecticut, HIV testing in, 87
Contact information, 115–116
Contact tracing programs, 89
Controversies, HIV/AIDS, 106–107
Cooper, Helene, 107
"The Coping and Change Study," 83
Cost
of drugs, 72
federal spending for HIV-related activities, according to agency, type of activity, 67t–68t
financing health care delivery, 59–61
health care delivery challenges, 61, 62, 63
of HIV/AIDS treatment, 66–71
of HIV/AIDS treatment, worldwide, 106–107
Ryan White CARE Act Title I grant awards, 69t
Ryan White CARE Act Title II grant awards, 70t
spending on AIDS research, 71
treatment research, 71
Counseling
home testing and, 90
post-HIV test counseling, 89
Court cases
Barton v. American Red Cross, 47
Faya v. Almarez, 66
Rossi v. Almarez, 66
Crixivan
reduction of virus loads with, 72
requirements for taking, 73–74
Cryptococcosis fungus, 18
Cunningham, W. E., 63
CXCR4 protein, 54
Cytomegalovirus
in late stage of HIV infection, 18
OI of HIV/AIDS, 9

D
Dale and Betty Bumpers Vaccine Research Center, 78
Davis, Brad, 80
De Jesus, Esteban, 80
Death
late stage of HIV infection and, 19
mortality from AIDS, 36–37
suicide, 84–86
Death benefits, 69–71

Morning-after treatment, 75
Mortality
    from AIDS, 36–37
    HIV/AIDS pandemic, death rates
        and, 98–99
    See also Death rates; Life expectancy
Mothers, HIV-infected
    babies born to, symptoms of, 49–50
    choice to bear children, 54
    in developing countries, 54
    diagnosis of HIV infection in
        children, 50–51
    HIV/AIDS in infants born to HIV-
        infected mothers, reported cases
        of, by selected characteristics, 38*t*
    HIV transmission in Europe, 102
    infants born to, 34
    nevirapine to reduce infection, 52
    perinatal infection, 51–52
    transmission of HIV, decrease in, 42
    See also Perinatal infection
MTM. *See* Male-to-male sexual contact
Mullis, Kary, 78
Multicenter AIDS Cohort Study, 16
Murex Diagnostics Inc., 22
Mycobacterium avium complex (MAC), 9
Mycobacterium tuberculosis
    tuberculosis caused by, 10
    worldwide TB, 99

N

Nabel, Gary, 78
Name-based case reporting, 87–89
Names, of organizations, 115–116
NAS (National Academy of Sciences), 41
NAs (nucleoside analogs), 52, 72–73
NASCAR, 80
NASCP (National AIDS/STD Control
    Program), 101
NASEN (North American Syringe
    Exchange Network), 94–95
NAT. *See* Nucleic acid test
National Academy of Sciences (NAS), 41
National Affordable Housing Act of
    1990, 84
National AIDS Housing Coalition, 84
National AIDS/STD Control Program
    (NASCP), 101
National Association of People with
    AIDS, 56–57
National Center for Health Statistics
    (NCHS), 117
National Commission on AIDS, 65
National Conference of State
    Legislatures, 92
*National Health Interview Survey in
    Advance Data* (National Center for
    Health Statistics), 117
National Institute of Allergy and
    Infectious Diseases (NIAID)
    discovery of fusin protein, 7

HIV vaccine and, 76
    vaccine efforts, 10–11
National Institute of Dental Research, 19
National Institutes of Health (NIH)
    condom use workshop, 92
    on dementia, 16
    spending on AIDS research, 71
    vaccine research center of, 78
"The National Multicenter AIDS Cohort
    Study," 83
*National Survey of Teens on HIV/AIDS,
    2000* (Kaiser Family Foundation), 110
NCAIDS (Chinese National Center for
    AIDS Prevention and Control), 21
NCHADS (Cambodian National Center
    for HIV/AIDS, Dermatology and
    STD), 103
NCHS (National Center for Health
    Statistics), 117
Needles
    HIV/AIDS prevention and, 91
    HIV transmission via, 19
    HIV transmission via IDU, 41
    needle exchange programs, 110
    needle safety for health care
        workers, 65
    prisoners and, 45–46
    syringe exchange programs, 93–95
    syringe exchange statistics, 95*t*
Netherlands, euthanasia in, 84
New England Journal of Medicine
    article on cost of treatment, 106
    article on costs of HIV patients, 59
    article on physician-assisted suicide,
        84–85, 118
    physicians and AIDS patients, 63
New York
    AIDS cases in, 25
    HIV testing of newborns in, 90
New York City, New York
    children with HIV in, 54–55
    survival time of AIDS patients in, 59
    Title I grants for, 67
New York Times, 107
Newborns, 90
    See also Infants
NIAID. *See* National Institute of Allergy
    and Infectious Diseases
NIH. *See* National Institutes of Health
*1993 Revised Classification for HIV
    Infection and Expanded AIDS
    Surveillance Case Definition for
    Adolescents and Adults* (Centers for
    Disease Control and Prevention)
    AIDS infection, clinical categories
        of, 15*t*
    classification system for HIV infection,
        expanded surveillance case
        definition for AIDS among
        adolescents and adults, 14*t*
    guidelines of, 13–14

1998 World Development Indicators (World
    Bank), 118
NNRTIs (nonnucleoside reverse
    transcriptase inhibitors), 52, 73
Noguer, Isabel, 102
Nonnucleoside reverse transcriptase
    inhibitors (NNRTIs), 52, 73
North American Syringe Exchange
    Network (NASEN), 94–95
North Carolina, 60
Nucleic acid test (NAT)
    for plasma screening, 20
    testing children for HIV, 49, 50
Nucleoside analogs (NAs), 52, 72–73
Nucleotide analogs, 73
Nureyev, Rudolf, 80
Nurses, 64
N.W.A. (Niggaz with Attitude), 80–81

O

O'Brien, Megan, 113
Office of National AIDS Policy, 59
Office visits
    of HIV/AIDS patients, 61–62
    number/percent of, by diagnostic/
        screening services ordered or
        provided, patient's sex, 62 (*t*6.1)
    number/percent of, by therapeutic/
        preventative services ordered or
        provided, patient's sex, 62 (*t*6.2)
OIs. *See* Opportunistic infections
Older people, with HIV/AIDS, 81–82
Olympic Games, 79–80
Opinion. *See* Public opinion
Opportunistic infections (OIs)
    in adults with AIDS, 49
    in HIV/AIDS progression, 8
    HIV development and, 9–10
    late stage of HIV infection and, 18
OraQuick Rapid HIV-1, 22
OraSure Technologies Inc., 22
Oregon
    "Death with Dignity Act," 84
    HIV testing in, 87
    physician-assisted suicide legalized in, 86
Organ transplants, 20
Organizations
    names, addresses of, 115–116
    resources on HIV/AIDS, 117–118
Origins, of HIV, 3–5
Orphans, from AIDS, 55
Outpatient treatment, 66
Oxford University, 5

P

Pacific Islanders. *See* Asian and Pacific
    Islander Americans
Pan-American Social Marketing
    Organization (PASMO), 107
Pang, Frederick F. Y., 90